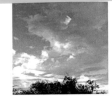

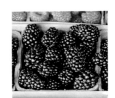

eating with grace

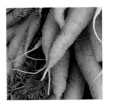

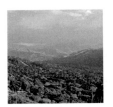

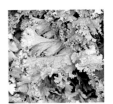

Eating With Grace: Learning to Feed Your Body and Nourish Your Life

For information, contact The Rev. W. Grace Nicodemus at 831.747.4222.

The content of this book is for general instruction only. Each person's physical, emotional, and spiritual condition is unique. The instruction in this book is not intended to replace or interrupt the reader's relationship with a physician or other professional. Please consult your doctor for matters pertaining to your specific health and diet.

To contact the publisher, visit
advancedhealthcoaching.com

To contact the co-author, visit
lcwcarmel@aol.com

Photographs: **Philip Geiger**
Cover and Interior Design: **Tessa Avila**
Copyediting: **Mary Barker**

ISBN-13: 978-1-5143-7887-8
ISBN-10: 1-5143-7887-6
Printed in the United States of America

eating with grace

learning to feed your body and nourish your life

W. GRACE NICODEMUS with **LISA CRAWFORD WATSON**

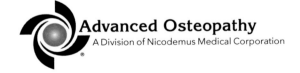

Advanced Osteopathy
A Division of Nicodemus Medical Corporation

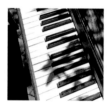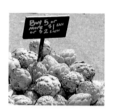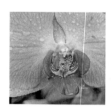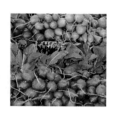

Contents

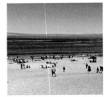
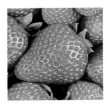

Acknowledgments

I thank God I found the courage to write this book. I thank Clarence L. Nicodemus, DO, PhD (a fully licensed physician in Neuromusculoskeletal Medicine, a specialty in Osteopathic Medicine) and my beloved husband, for giving me the love and support that has enabled me to see myself through compassionate eyes, and to believe I should write this book. I thank my children, Nola and Scott, who have been, since early on, my reasons to continue to live and to succeed.

I am grateful to Marilyn Manning, M.A., Ed.D., for her training in neurolinguistic programming; the late Dr. Virginia Satir, for her work through PAIRS (Practical Application of Intimate Relationship Skills); and applied neuroscience specialist Nancy White, Ph.D. and Pat Farley, MA, for their wise counsel and progressive approaches to emotional recovery and development.

I want to acknowledge Nina Quartaro for her friendship and support throughout the years. She and I met over our eating issues in the early '80s, and bonded over lunch. We have been together through the ups and downs of our lives, forging a friendship that has brought her closer to me than family.

I also want to recognize Monya Gray-Scherzer for her love and support, and her willingness to see me through all the revelations during ministerial school. She saw through my fears and other feelings to figure out who I really was and foster who I could become.

I thank the principals at the Institute for Integrative Nutrition® (IIN), for giving me the tools and the truth about eating well and living healthier, so I could mend my heart,

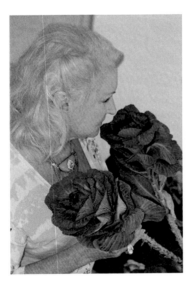

my mind and my body in preparation for writing this book. Their research and wisdom provided the basis for the programs I present to patients, clients, friends and family, and now you, my readers, who have endured enough heartbreak and held onto enough hope to wonder what I have to say.

I thank my colleague, Chef Paola Mikes, who completes our health coaching team, for showing me that healthy food can taste good, feel satisfying, and nourish my body. Rather than just "giving me a fish to feed me for a day," she has taught me "how to fish"—how to shop for, prepare, and serve nutritious meals, "that I may feed myself for a lifetime."

I thank author Lisa Crawford Watson for putting my experiences, my thoughts and feelings, my training and my wisdom into words, so I could share them with kindred spirits. I thank Mary Barker for her insightful editing. I thank graphic designer Tessa Avila for her artistic vision in giving shape and form to this book, and photographer Philip Geiger for adding a thousand words of poetry with every picture.

Most of all, I thank you, dear reader, for taking this journey with me toward recovery and a happier, healthier life.

To anyone who has struggled with food issues,
this book is for you.

Introduction

It was New Year's Eve 1999, and everyone in the ballroom of the Embassy Suites hotel was dressed to dine, to dance, to celebrate the advent of a new century. I glanced across this room filled with sequins and silk, and took in the crowd. Everyone was up and on their feet, pressed closely to one another, listening to the band, arms overhead, hips gyrating, and toes tapping, dancing in tight circles where they stood. Except for one woman, who listened to the music without moving. I recognized her as a local nutritionist and fitness trainer, an exceptionally fit woman with the figure of a young athlete. With admiration, I looked at her long, naturally curly hair, and the satin slip of a gown that skimmed her lean frame.

What stood out most to me about this attractive woman was that she wasn't enjoying herself. Her *self*. Instead of getting lost in the music and dancing her joy, she was looking around, studying the appearance of others, and glancing, now and then, at herself. Repeatedly, she adjusted her dress and pressed her hand against her stomach, smoothing the soft fabric as if to hide something that wasn't there.

Just before I returned my attention to the music and the magic of New Year's Eve, I thought, "Is anyone safe from the issues of body image, insecurity and self-worth?"

I believe I actually know a few people who are. I had a girlfriend in school who ate a second helping of spaghetti because it tasted so good, who exercised because it was fun, and who wore clothes because they were comfortable or colorful or clean—not because they could hide her indiscretions. I had a friend who loved dessert, so she ate hers very slowly, in tiny bites, savoring each morsel, while another chose to "slam it down" and serve herself a second slice.

But I also have a friend, a consummate athlete, who trains every day and competes regularly in running and cycling, who eats what she wants and has a lean, muscled body. I envied her until I learned that she has bulimia, purging at the end of the day, whatever she has consumed that has not been metabolized by all her activity. Then she sinks to the floor by the toilet bowl, and sobs.

All of these people, mostly women but not all, are tortured by their relationship with food and the self-loathing they carry with them. They are so consumed by guilt, grief, fear, disappointment, anger, angst, they are missing out on their lives, on the joys of just being alive. I know these women, intimately, for I am one of them.

What I realize is that even the seemingly most successful, confident people often harbor their own private tortures and traumas around eating, gaining weight, and dieting. Can someone be successful and fat, sexy and fat, happy and fat? This has to stop. We deserve better. I read somewhere that America's obsession with food and weight is our very own private terrorism, threatening our confidence, our sense of security and our productivity in this nation.

This has to stop. We deserve better.

For me, the torture came at the fanciest party of the year. I remember it as if it were last night because I've replayed it in my mind so many times, keeping it close and the pain, acute. It was a black-tie fundraiser, a rare opportunity to dress up and dance the night away. For weeks I had known what I was going to wear—my satin ball gown, a halter dress "cut down to there," kind of like Marilyn Monroe over the subway grate, only in red. The back was low, the shoes were high, and I imagined slipping into the satin and spinning around until my skirt flared and I, Wilma Grace, had become as fabulous as Norma Jean.

The afternoon of the event, I had my hair done in something sophisticated. I did my own makeup with a bit of evening elegance. I slid my gown off its hanger and pressed the dress to my body in front of the mirror, admiring. It had been two years since I'd worn it, on another night to remember, and I was looking forward to feeling the same magic.

I tucked my head into the halter, let the dress drop down my body, and reached behind to pull up the zipper.

It wasn't that the dress was a bit tight, that I would have to stuff myself into spandex, never take a deep breath, and forgo food for the night, as I had done so many times before. This time, to my horror, the sides of the zipper didn't even meet.

I let the dress drop to the floor and then sank down into yards of satin and self-loathing. Then I called my friends and told them I'd come down with the flu, and would have to skip the evening. I knew they, too, had spent weeks anticipating and hours getting ready. I knew some of them would not go without me. In a move both utterly confounding and completely understandable, I soothed myself with a box of chocolates.

The next morning, my good friend said, "Why didn't you just pick something else to wear?"

But you see, that would have required self-confidence, self-esteem, and a willingness to accept myself regardless of my weight.

And I will tell you something. We can gather all the information in the world about eating well in the interest of healthy living. But if we don't value ourselves, if something about the way we were fed food or information about ourselves as a child has negatively affected our self-esteem, we may not know our worth. And if we don't believe our body deserves to be healthy and fit, we may not see the point of feeding ourselves well.

So any of you who have ever been traumatized by your own body image, from living overweight or under weight, or vacillating between the two; any of you who have, therefore, lifted yourself out of the opportunity to participate in a joyful, productive life, this book is for you. If you are weary of dealing with shame, anger, disappointment, judgment, frustration, rage or fear you have experienced from your eating and its effects, if you want to clear away the emotional wreckage of your life that has led to your emotional relationship to food, read on.

Perhaps it's time to shield your eyes from the glint of the social mirror, to broaden your perspective and see your past through a loving, caring, completely clear lens. Understand you made the best decisions you could with the tools and information you had at the time. And know, with new information and new tools, you can make new decisions about who you are, what you deserve, and where you want to go. It is time to look toward your future with confidence, presence, self-awareness, peace, and the anticipation of a healthy, happy, engaged life.

For starters, you need to understand that it's not your fault. Not completely, anyway. If you feel your weight gain is the result of not exercising your willpower, of not pushing yourself away from the table, not grabbing another handful of chocolates; understand you've been up against a pretty powerful opponent. Sugar. More addictive than crack and infinitely more acceptable, we are now realizing it's in just about everything, and it's a secret weapon against our waistlines. Particularly when we're using it to soothe our souls.

I had fought the food war for so many years in so many ways, and I lost the battle every time. Not until I was introduced to the Institute for Integrative Nutrition®, not until I enrolled in the Institute, not until I learned what the largest nutrition school in the country has to say about diet and nutrition, and what it truly means to nourish ourselves, did I understand how to coach myself and my clients, into a better relationship with ourselves and with food. I have heard countless stories from clients and friends about experiences that have contributed to their struggles to achieve and maintain a healthy weight. I wish I had room to share them all with you. Rest assured, you are not alone in this. I didn't know if I had the courage to tell my own story, to shed the mask I had so carefully constructed through well-cut clothes, fabulous shoes and accessories designed to distract, to draw attention only to the part of me I was willing to present. The facade.

And then it hit me. Authenticity—or the lack of it—is one of our biggest roadblocks in our journey toward self-discovery, toward healing, toward recovery. We need to be honest with ourselves and with others, just as we need the food industry to come clean with us about what goes into our food. I figure if I can share a few of my truths, you'll find a way to get at yours, and maybe we'll inspire positive, life-affirming change in ourselves and in others.

After achieving my own success by realizing I'm worth it, by making better choices, by eating well to reach a healthy weight, and by maintaining it, I felt inspired to help others do the same. In 2014, I established Advanced Health Coaching (AHC) in Monterey, CA. As a health coach, I am an advocate for living an energized and passionate life. Through AHC, I work with my clients to help them create happy, healthy lives through a flexible approach, free from denial and strict discipline. By working together, we discover the food and lifestyle choices that best support them, knowing that making gradual, lifelong changes will enable them to reach their current and future health goals.

While this may not be the definitive book on learning how to nourish ourselves, it explores the journey of one woman, and many like me, who have found a way out of the dark as we learn enough to see the clearing. This has worked for me, it has worked for my clients, and it can work for you. My goal is to help my clients and, now, you, discover your own approach to healthy eating for healthy living.

We've been told by many that knowledge is power. But if you've ever done something you knew you shouldn't, you know it sometimes takes more than knowledge to do what's best. I am neither a doctor nor an expert on nutrition. But I am an expert on my own trials and triumphs, and I have learned through experience, and training by the Institute of Integrative Nutrition® how to achieve a healthy life.

So permit me to share the wisdom I've learned along the way. Try the exercises at the end of each chapter, (which I still practice), making sure you have a coach, counselor, minister or trusted friend available to discuss and help you make sense of your outcomes and feelings. Indulge yourself in the beautiful photographs of all that nourishes us, and try Chef Paola Mikes' healthy and delicious recipes sprinkled throughout these pages. See if you can find a kindred spirit in me and a guiding light in my book.

~ Rev. W. Grace Nicodemus

Cilantro and Lime Shrimp Tacos

SLAW INGREDIENTS

¼ medium green cabbage,
   thinly sliced

½ small purple cabbage,
   very thinly sliced

½ cup shredded carrots

¼ cup real organic mayonnaise

¼ cup coconut milk

2 tsp honey

1 tbsp raw apple cider vinegar

¼ tsp salt

TACO INGREDIENTS

2 tbsp coconut oil

1 ½ lb wild-caught shrimp, peeled
   and deveined, tails removed

1 tbsp minced garlic

1 tsp paprika

1 tsp chili powder

2 tbsp fresh lime juice

3 tbsp fresh cilantro

Salt & pepper to taste

A quick, easy, light, savory summer supper

DIRECTIONS

Slaw: Combine shredded cabbage and carrots in bowl. In separate bowl, mix milk, mayonnaise, vinegar, honey and salt. Pour over cabbage. Toss to combine. Cover and refrigerate for a couple of hours.

Shrimp: In medium bowl, mix shrimp, spices, lemon juice, and salt and pepper. Heat coconut oil in heavy skillet over high heat. Add shrimp and toss, cooking until pink and opaque. Remove from heat, add cilantro, and set aside.

EXTRAS

whole corn tortillas, warmed • pico de gallo • guacamole • lime wedges • sour cream

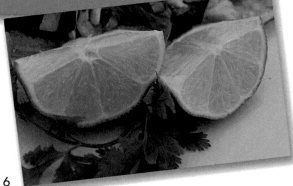

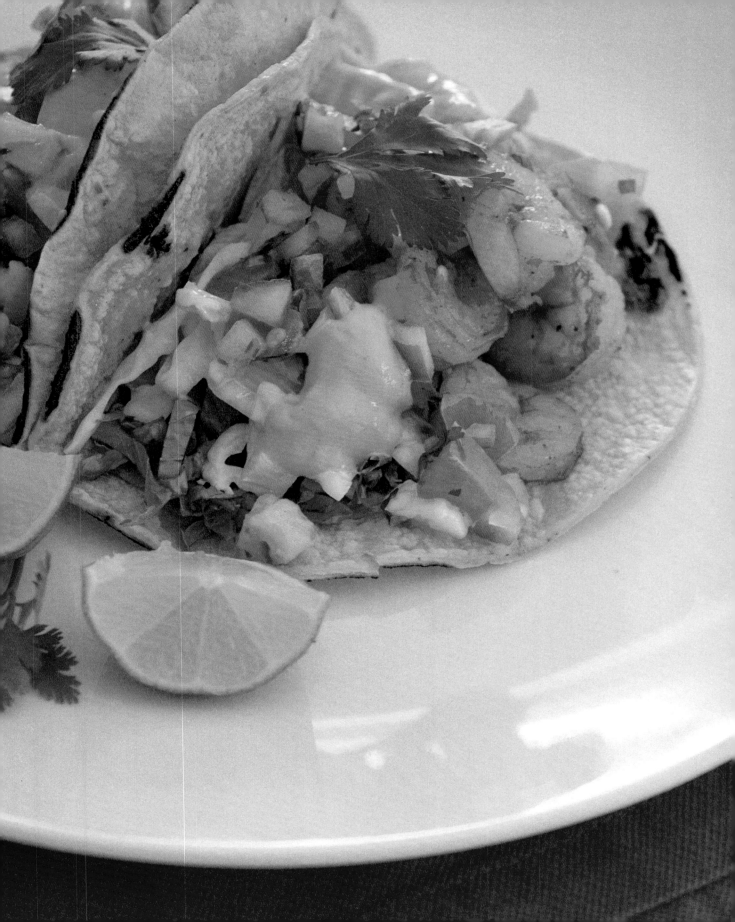

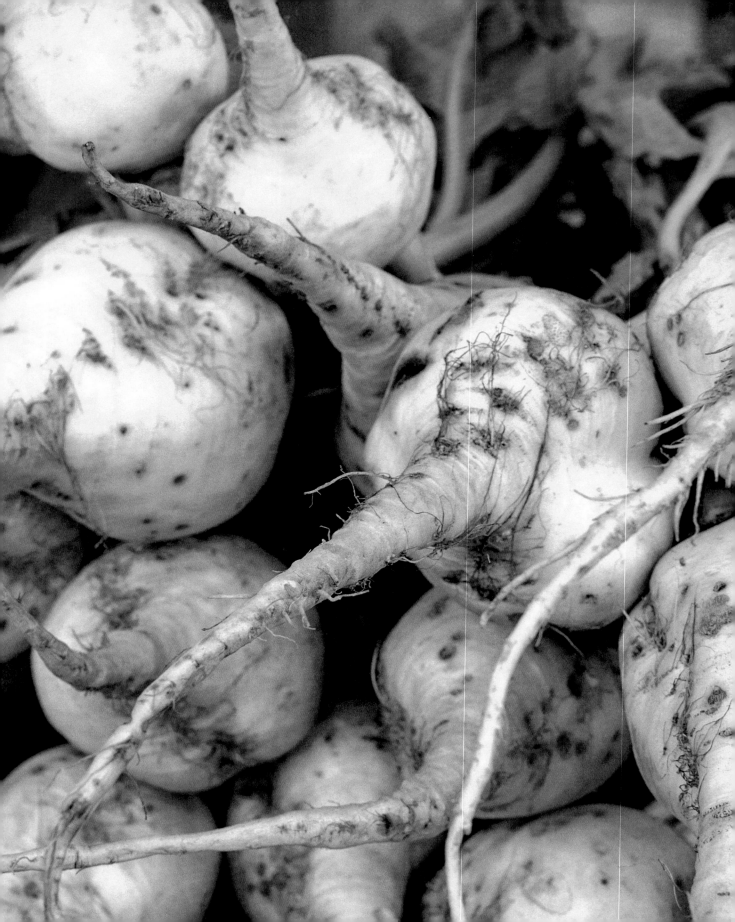

1

Rough Start

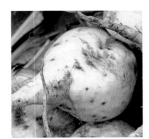 A month before I was born in the summer of '42, my mother, flush with expectancy, opened the front door to receive two, full-dress naval officers, bearing a telegram from the U.S. Department of the Navy. My father, Navy fighter pilot William H. Warden, had gone missing in action in the Battle of Midway during WWII. The day before, my mother was busily preparing her nursery and her life for the much-anticipated return of her young husband, and the arrival of William H. Warden, Jr., their son. Upon reading the news that my father was missing, my mother collected her coat and her handbag, and went to the wrong side of town to attempt an abortion.

Mother drove to the address she had scrawled on the back of an envelope, and climbed the wood stairs tacked onto the weathered-white siding that led her to a room above a garage. Inside the spare space, she saw a table in the middle of the room beneath a naked light bulb shining like a spotlight on the stained surface of the wood. She climbed onto the table and waited to have her life restored by eliminating another. Instead, she was told she was too far along in her pregnancy to go ahead with an abortion. So she slid down from the table and slunk down the stairs to the security of her car.

My mother ultimately forgoing the abortion had nothing to do with preserving me. Believing her dreams had died with her husband, she simply wasn't about to go with them.

One month later, on June 17, my mother received the only possible news that could have been worse. "It's a girl!" Believing the last thing she wanted in her circumstance was a baby, she found she was wrong. The last thing she wanted was a girl. In the absence of her husband, the only person she likely had ever or would ever truly love, she had settled on the idea of an heir, a symbol and reminder of her beloved, in little William.

And that is how I came to be named Wilma. The symbol and reminder of everything that went wrong in my mother's life. She was stuck with me, and I was stuck with the knowledge that she had tried to get rid of me. When she couldn't, she had prayed for a boy to be named for my father. I knew this because she told me. All the time.

This woeful welcome into the world set the tone for my life. My mother's desperate disappointment colored the myopic lens through which I looked at life, altering my perspective as I tried to make sense of my world. My mother was larger than life, and everything she said was true. As a child, I had no other experience, no context in which to believe otherwise. And no words to tell her how it felt.

As it turned out, my father had not been killed in the Pacific Theater. After his squadron launched off the Enterprise aircraft carrier, he was shot down and presumed lost at sea. Severely injured, with a bullet that would remain lodged in the right side of his head for the rest of his life, my father spent a week tucked inside a rubber raft, desperately trying to reach land. One month later, he did, and was discovered by a Catholic monk, Father Emery, who lay my father upon a canvas stretcher, piled high with food and other supplies, to ferry him, unnoticed, across enemy lines.

And so Dad came home. I was 9 months old when we met, and my earliest memory tells me I found love in his eyes.

As I grew older, I got what he saw in my mother. She had fiery red hair and the temperament that went with it which, I suppose, could be seductive. At least at first. Dad met her at a popular bar in Florida, a flashy young gal with a quick wit, a sharp tongue, and a figure like Jane Russell. In those days, a divorced cocktail waitress with two kids worked overtime to seduce a man into saving her life. My father was smitten.

In a different story, I might have been the adored child of star-crossed lovers, who got their happy ending. But I was born to a woman who didn't want me, and a man who often wasn't there.

Was this the beginning of my illicit love affair with food, the most tantalizing yet tortured relationship I would ever experience? Absolutely. It was the beginning of everything, the launch of my life, and the start of my most lasting relationship, one that would endure long after my parents had passed.

As I've grown older, and my lifeline rather long, I have imagined myself, more than once, ready to tell my parents what I've thought of his disappearances and her overt disappointment, utter disregard, and often impossible expectations that left me damned if I complied and damned if I didn't. But each time I've stopped, with pen hovering over paper, believing my parents wouldn't understand what they did or didn't, wouldn't comprehend the impact on me, and wouldn't have any idea what to do about it.

Moreover, part of the beauty of age and experience is the wisdom and compassion we develop for those who have gone before us. In my experiences as a wife, a mother, an adult, I have come to realize that my mother had her own struggles, her own hard moments. I understand, now, that she raised her children as she was raised. She simply was doing the best she knew how.

Now that my parents are gone, I realize this letter isn't about them. It's about me, about working through my own feelings, by putting them into words and, through that exercise, learning how I might shed the emotional baggage that has kept me from enjoying my God-given life and my right to make the most of it.

Goal

Give yourself the freedom that comes from forgiving others
and, perhaps, yourself.

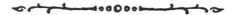

PART ONE   Assess your emotional wounds as a way to gather your thoughts for the letter you will write to those who inflicted the pain. You will write this letter, but you will not send or give it to the person to whom it is addressed.

Step One   Think of a time when someone criticized or spoke unkindly to you. As you took in those words, along with your emotional reaction, where in your body did you feel the pain or discomfort? Was it your shoulders, your belly, your heart, hips, hands, legs, feet?

Step Two   Using the terms below and the chart on the next page, take inventory of the episodes when you have felt emotionally wounded. Did it affect your:

P   Pride

S   Safety

SE   Self Esteem

SC   Self Confidence

SI   Self Image

J   Joy

SX   Sexuality

Step Three   Make a list of those you need to forgive to help yourself move on. Don't forget to include yourself on the list where appropriate.

Step Four   Fill in the table on page 13 in preparation for the letter(s) you will write.

Year or your age at time of incident	Name of person or institution	What was said or done to you?	How did this affect you?	Whom do you need to forgive?
Age 20	Natalie	"Run harder" fatty / porky	P, SE, SC, SI	Natalie

13

PART TWO   The Letter(s)

Step One   Referring to your inventory, handwrite a letter to each person or organization from which you felt hurt. Include the following information:

1. Date
2. Person or institution
3. What was done or said to you
4. How it affected you
5. Whom you need to forgive

Step Two   Describe, in as much detail as you can, every hurt, angry slur, disappointment, misstatement and judgment you received from yourself or from others about your weight.

Step Three   Using your iPhone or other device, record your letter as you read it aloud. Play it back to yourself and, as it plays, tear a page out of an old phonebook or notebook, wad it up into a ball, and throw it into a pile, calling out the name of the person or institution that hurt you. Throw hard and with passion. The more physical you can be in doing this exercise, the more you will release any pent-up emotional baggage from the past.

Step Four   Look at the pile and witness how much emotional baggage you have released. Feel the empty emotional space it has left behind.

Step Five   Now is the time to fill up that space with forgiveness for yourself and others. In most cases, their words and actions have come from their own internal wounds, and they did not realize the damage they were doing. Remember, as renowned author Anne Lamott says, "Not forgiving is like drinking rat poison and then waiting for the rat to die."

Forgiving yourself will set you free, enabling you to see yourself as you truly are—healthy, happy and ready to start living the joyful, productive life of which you have always dreamed.

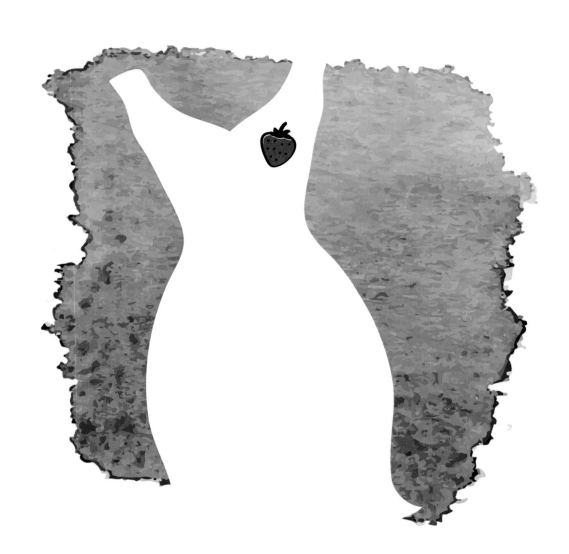

GRANOLA INGREDIENTS

½ cup chopped almonds

½ cup almond flour

3 cups old-fashioned oats

½ cup shaved coconut

½ tsp salt

⅓ cup honey

⅓ cup coconut sugar

3 tbsp coconut oil

½ tsp vanilla extract

½ tsp almond extract

PARFAIT INGREDIENTS

½ cup almond coconut granola

¼ cup strawberries

¼ cup blueberries

¼ cup blackberries

6 oz vanilla coconut yogurt

Almond Coconut Honey Granola

Fresh, fruity, and creamy . . .
like having dessert for breakfast

DIRECTIONS

Preheat oven to 350 degrees.

Chop almonds coarsely, and pour into large bowl. Pour oats, coconut, salt, and coconut sugar into bowl, and stir to combine. In small saucepan, combine honey and coconut oil. Heat for 1 to 2 minutes, just to dissolve coconut oil. Remove from heat, and add vanilla and almond extract.

Pour honey mixture over oats, and stir until evenly coated. Pour oats evenly onto Silpat nonstick baking sheet or parchment-lined baking sheet. Bake oats for 15 minutes, and then stir them around. Return them to oven for 5 more minutes. Remove from oven and let cool. After completely cool, break the granola into clusters and store in an airtight container.

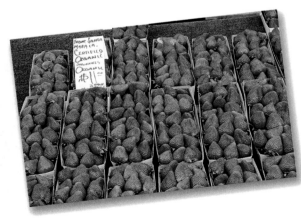

Breakfast Parfait

DIRECTIONS

Layer berries, yogurt, and granola in clear glass. Serve immediately. Enjoy.

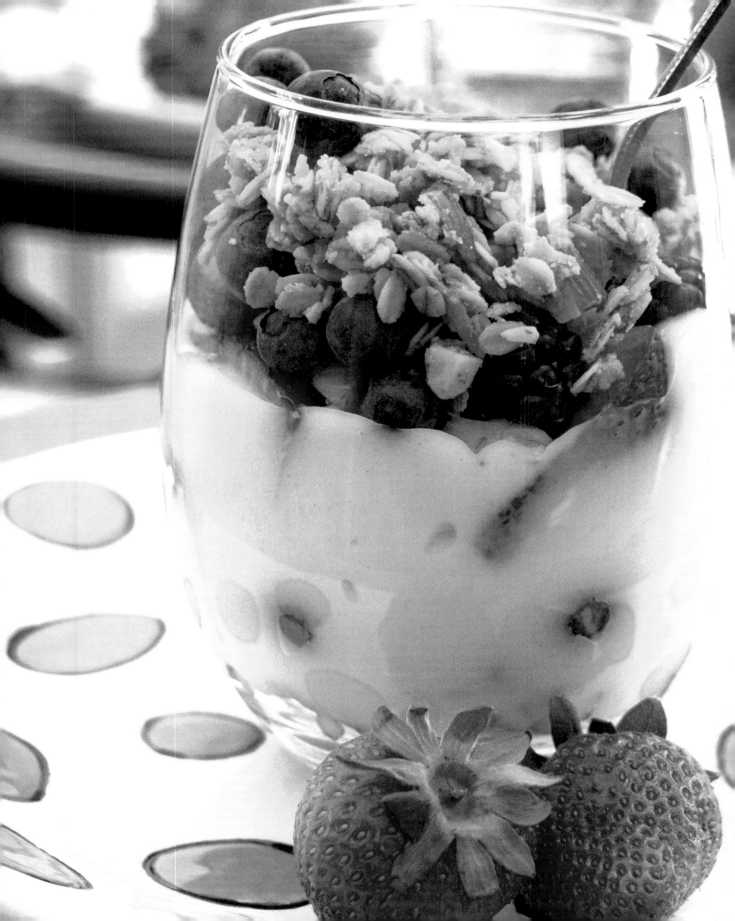

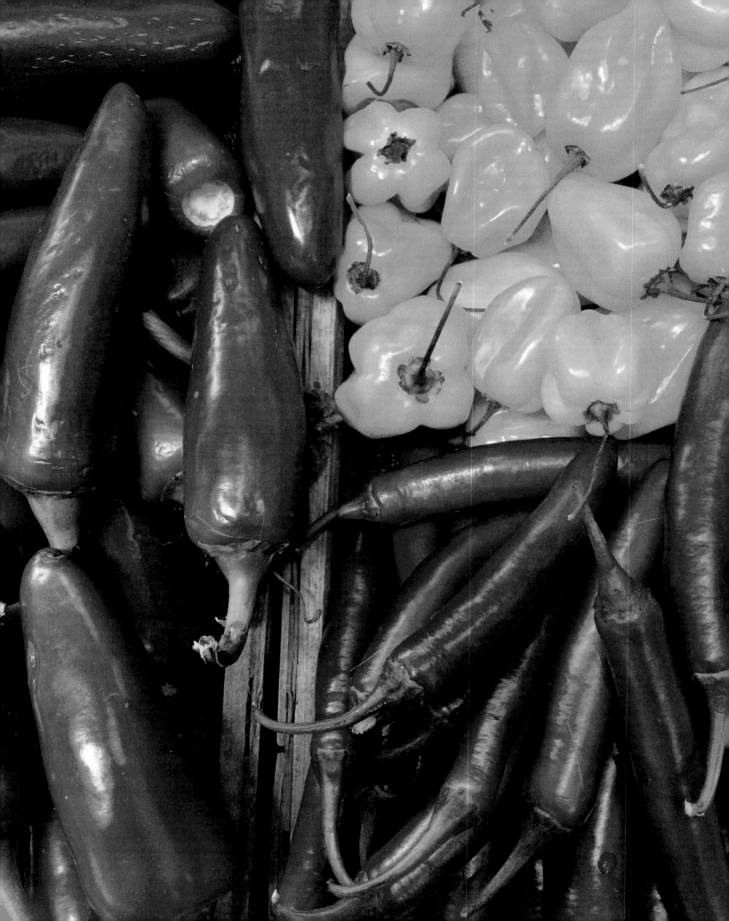

2

Marching to the Beat

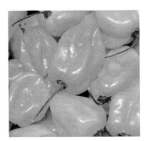

I liked the way the fabric felt, soft and smooth between my thumb and forefinger, as I pulled it up my body and shimmied into the skimpy little uniform with the cap sleeves and skater skirt. I liked even better how it skimmed my body, making my waist look small, and helping me feel sleek and strong, and maybe even a little sexy.

Pretty wasn't an option, my mother would remind me every time I twirled in front of the mirror, seeking her approval. But sexy, she said, now that could get a woman what she wanted.

Mostly, I liked how my uniform said I'd made it in this world. I had what it took. I was a majorette, fit to strut my stuff in front of everybody. Or at least the Coronado High School Marching Band, spinning that baton like it was on fire. Sometimes, it was.

The popular girls, with their long legs and corn-silk hair, were cheerleaders, pompon girls and homecoming queens. They were the *in* crowd, setting the standard for beautiful, desirable, cool. Majorettes were on the fringe of that. But in the band, we were royalty.

My older half sister, Yvonne, with her French name, tall, slender body and big attitude, was a majorette. And so it became my mission to become one, too, if only to prove that a regular girl named Wilma Warden could someday even make *head* majorette, mostly because Yvonne would not.

Yvonne said my tryout, in contemporary language, sucked, and I only made the majorette corps my freshman year because I was her sister. Yet there I was, prancing and spinning. And mostly hoping Yvonne's behavior wouldn't hurt my chances after she ran off at 16, and her reputation was the only thing that came home. Still, her words put doubt in my mind, and reminded me that my thighs were a little fuller than most everyone else's.

While I was in high school, Marilyn Monroe came to our hometown of Coronado, CA to film "Some Like It Hot" at the Hotel del Coronado. In the part she was filming, as I watched from the deck of the hotel, she was to run from the hotel, down across the sand, to the shore. What I remember most besides her blonde hair and electric beauty, is that she was not slim—not by the norms of 1959, and certainly not by today's standards. And I remember thinking I was no bigger than she was. For a moment, I wondered if there was more to sexy than size.

One afternoon, I slipped into my uniform and stamped into my short, white boots covered in rabbit fur that fluttered when we marched, and went to one of our first flag-and-baton practices of the season. I was so proud, exhilarated, really, as I took my place in line, twirled a horizontal figure eight, and spun that silver pipe into the air. I could feel my heart pounding as I caught it and kept the twirl going, literally, without missing a beat.

After practice, some of the kids invited me to go with them into San Diego. I knew I was not allowed to leave Coronado Island without my parents, but my excitement at being included overrode my better judgment, and I went along. I can still remember the giddy feelings of freedom and independence as I pranced down the street with my friends, ordered my own Coca-Cola®, and sat next to what had to be one of the loveliest boys in school.

By the time the car full of kids pulled up in front of my house, I was pretty sure that boy was getting ready to ask for my number. I opened the car door but paused ever so briefly before getting out, glancing back at him with a shy smile. His eyes darkened and his mouth dropped as my mother rushed through the front door and across the lawn. Yanking me out of the car by my hair, she threw me to the ground and then beat me with my metal flag until it broke. Then she tore off my beloved uniform, stripping me of so much more than my identity as my friends watched, in silence.

Once my mother relented, I got up and ran, tripping and then scrambling ahead of her into the house. I never saw my friends leave, and I never heard from that boy.

My mother followed me inside and resumed her beating with anything she could reach until she had exhausted her anger. As she walked away, she threw my tattered uniform at me and said, "Go eat something. You'll feel better."

I chose a mayonnaise sandwich on white bread with extra sugar, and washed down my despair with a soda.

I was too bruised to dress for P.E., but my mother forced me to go to school. Afterward, I came straight home every day, restricted from extracurricular activities for a year. I spent most of that time eating, but my mother was wrong. I never did feel better. More than anything, the food tasted tragic, lonely, and desperately sad. And yet still, I ate, finding strange comfort in the chewing, while I swallowed her dismissive messages whole.

My mother did mend my majorette uniform, making it tighter and shorter than before, just to expose my shame.

It's amazing to me that I continued performing throughout high school, despite my damaged sense of self-worth. Except I believe being a majorette was my life support all the way to head majorette. It wasn't the first beating I had endured, and it certainly wasn't the last. But it was among the more memorable. It introduced me to the concept of comfort food and widened my waist as it whittled away my self-esteem, yet it somehow motivated me to become one bold baton twirler.

So many years later, when I look at myself smiling in the lineup of majorettes in that faded photo in my high school yearbook, I realize I was not a big girl. But the images engraved in my memory and my truth at the time reflected what I was taught, by my mother, my sister, the cheerleaders and Audrey Hepburn, Kim Novak, Doris Day. I was fat. While thin, my unobtainable ideal, was all that mattered.

I have lived decades beyond those formative years, in which my sense of self was so firmly established. So it still amazes me how well it has withstood the passage of time and training and maturing. For years, it undergirded the decisions I made about myself, and supported my heroic efforts to diet myself to impossibly thin or to feed my feelings until, by the time I was a young adult, I was dangerously overweight.

Truthfully, even then, I didn't know what to do. I desperately wanted out of the claustrophobic, burden of my body that imprisoned or maybe protected me from participating in a joyful, productive life. I've often wondered how obese people get anything done.

I moved slowly, felt uncomfortable in my skin, my bulk, my clothes, my chair. And I thought of very little else. How could I be so hungry when I was already so fat?

I later learned that not everyone who is overweight is upset about it. Not everyone above a size 10 or 12 sees themselves as overweight. Not everyone who believes they should lose weight takes it personally. That was big for me. Huge. Unconditional love.

Being defined by something other than weight or appearance. I imagined how freeing that must feel, and how it could pull me up and out from under the burden of weight and allow me to address it as a benevolent friend.

Imagine.

Goal

Gain insight into the interaction and communication styles
among family members during mealtimes,
and the effect this may have had on you.
What messages did you get about mealtime and food?

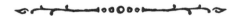

PART ONE

Step One   On a blank piece of paper, draw a picture of your kitchen counter, dining room table or TV trays where you, as a young person, ate most of your meals with the members of your household. See the diagram on page 24.

Step Two   Draw a patterned line from one chair to another, indicating who was most likely to speak to whom and in what tone. Make a note along each line where there was anger, discord, disagreement, or violence during the meal.

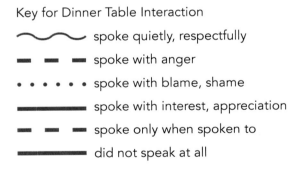

Key for Dinner Table Interaction

〰〰〰 spoke quietly, respectfully

▬ ▬ ▬ spoke with anger

• • • • • spoke with blame, shame

▬▬▬▬▬ spoke with interest, appreciation

▬ ▬ ▬ spoke only when spoken to

▬▬▬▬▬ did not speak at all

Use the same key, whether you dined together at a table or gathered, using TV trays or your laps.

Step Three   Write the name of the person in each seat. Notice what part you played in the dialogue or interaction. Were you quiet, conversant, outspoken, unkind? Were you ignored, engaged, criticized or hit during dinner?

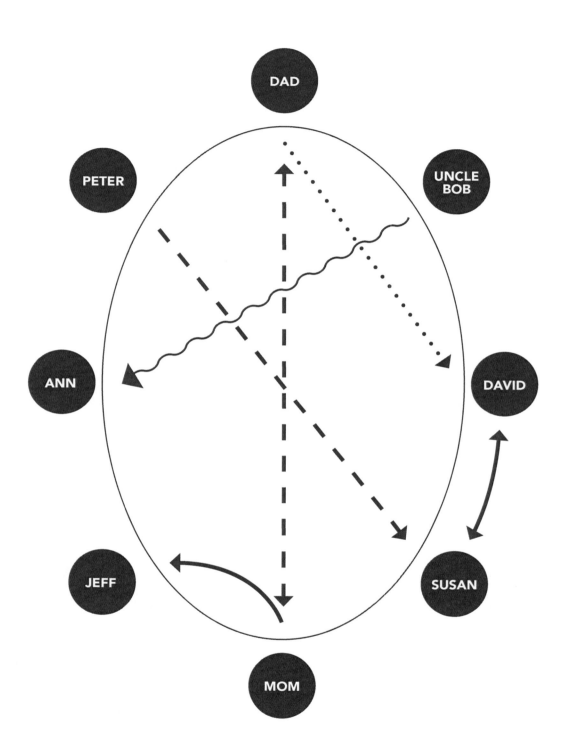

PART TWO

Step One   Write what you remember about your childhood experiences at mealtimes and what comes up for you. Did you say grace before eating? Were your mealtimes joyful or unpleasant? Stressed or relaxed? Was the conversation respectful and engaged or disrespectful and disregarded? Did you attempt to protect someone, or did someone protect you? Was money talked about in terms of how much the food cost? Did you feel a connection between the cost of food and how much you ate? Where were you in the dynamic, and how did you feel about it?

Step Two   Add a discussion on what happens and how you feel about your experiences at mealtime, now. How is it similar or different, and why?

Step Three   Read to yourself what you have written, mindful of what feelings arise in you. Allow yourself to be more curious than condemning as you make decisions about how you want to feel and what you want to experience at mealtimes, now. As your awareness shifts, so too, will your responses. Notice how other members in your household respond via how they communicate with each other and with you.

Zucchini Noodle Lasagna

INGREDIENTS

1 lb ground beef (grass fed)
    or ground turkey
1 cup onion, chopped
3 cloves garlic, minced
1 tbsp chopped fresh basil
3 tbsp fresh parsley
1 tsp chopped fresh oregano
1 tsp chopped fresh thyme
4 zucchini, sliced thinly
1 8-oz box of mushrooms, sliced
2 jars marinara sauce
16 oz full-fat ricotta cheese
2 cups mozzarella cheese
2 tbsp olive oil
Salt and pepper, to taste

*A hearty—but not heavy—
alternative to traditional lasagna*

DIRECTIONS

Preheat oven to 375 degrees.

Brown ground beef with olive oil in large pot over medium heat, stirring frequently. Add in garlic, mushrooms, onion. and continue to sauté for 5 minutes.

Stir in marinara sauce and herbs. Bring sauce to boil, then reduce heat to medium and simmer for 30 min. Remove from heat and set aside.

Meanwhile, slice zucchini into ⅛" slices, lightly salt, and set aside for 10 minutes. Zucchini has a lot of water when cooked, but salting it takes out a lot of moisture. After 10 minutes, blot excess moisture with a paper towel.

To make cheese mixture, in a bowl combine ricotta cheese, mozzarella, 1 tbsp parsley, and salt & pepper to taste. Mix well.

Place a layer of sauce in baking dish and layer zucchini over sauce, followed by cheese mixture. Repeat, alternating a layer of sauce, then zucchini, and finish with a layer of mozzarella cheese on top.

Bake lasagna, covered with foil, at 375°F for 25 minutes. Remove foil and bake for an additional 15 minutes. Cool for 10 minutes before serving.

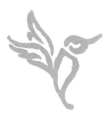

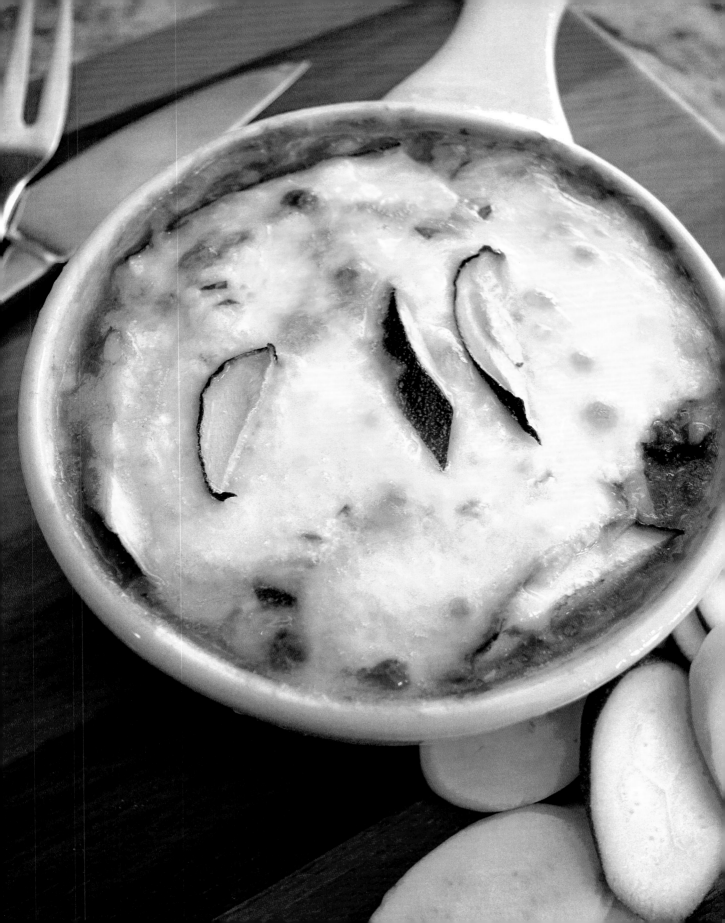

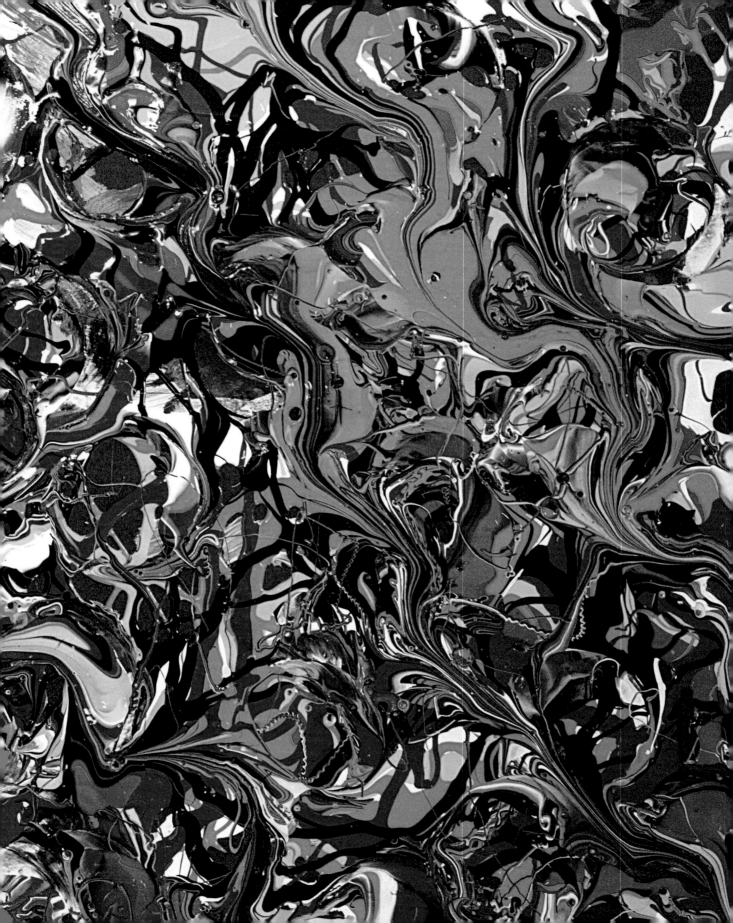

3

Down the Aisle

As a child, my weight was determined by what my mother served, and her insistence that I clean my plate. Once I grew up, my weight was determined by my social life. I was the queen of "date weight." Whether I was getting out of a relationship or looking to get into one, I had mastered the art of getting my weight down low enough to be devastating in my departure, or drop-dead gorgeous upon arrival. Which actually makes sense since I was metaphorically killing myself to get into skinny jeans that looked as good in the "walk away" as they had in the approach. My diet strategy was "dating." As long as I was single, I didn't eat.

I had plenty of opportunities to perfect this.

However, when I was comfortably ensconced in a relationship; happy, secure, and cooking as if I were Southern, I tended to pack on the weight with the permission of a holiday season, year round. Every bite of crispy, crunchy, chewy, nutty, chocolaty indulgence was worth it, until I finished chewing and swallowed my indiscretion.

And this is how it came to pass that, two years after I slipped into my lace wedding dress with the narrow waist and nothing-to-hide silhouette, I tipped the scales at 207 pounds. In my wedded bliss, I had perfected the art of "fat and happy," except not happy. In my desperation to do something other than divorce my husband to become thin again, I went online and discovered the Rader Programs.

Their message spoke to me: "At Rader Programs, we want to assure the millions of individuals suffering from eating disorders like anorexia, compulsive overeating and bulimia of three vital facts:

It's not your fault.

You are not alone.

We can help.

"We understand that eating disorders are controlling your life, and they've made food the centerpiece of your existence. We are well-acquainted with the feelings of isolation, depression, guilt and shame that you are experiencing. Whether your eating disorder causes you to starve yourself, excessively exercise, abuse substances, or binge and purge, there is a common truth: you are struggling with a dangerous disorder that, if left untreated, could be fatal.

"However, we know from experience that freedom from eating disorders and a lifetime of recovery can be achieved. The cornerstone of our philosophy is that your recovery depends upon recognizing the underlying causes of your eating disorder and, with professional guidance, taking action to facilitate necessary lifestyle changes."

I was the person who ate because I was happy, because I was sad, and sometimes, because I was hungry. I ate when I was in pain or feeling frustrated, when I was filled with anger, fear or hope. I ate my meals in the car between business appointments, focused not on the food—how it tasted, felt, filled me up—but on the road. When I got home, it seemed as if I hadn't eaten. And so I would. Again.

For awhile, I joined a group of female friends, who met once a week for drinks. I'd order something sexy in a stem and sip it slowly, but I wouldn't order any food. I figured the liquor was plenty of calories for the night. And still, I gained weight, not understanding why. I remember one night, dressing in a beautiful navy-and-white two-piece suit, excited to gussy up and go out on the town with my friends. But all evening, the suit jacket kept gaping; I had become too big for it. It was all I thought about, besides wondering how quickly I could slip out of the club, out of that suit, and into my shame, alone.

The following week, I enrolled myself in the Rader Institute at Intracare Hospital in Houston, and sent myself to a one-week rehab for compulsive overeaters. My husband drove me there and visited during the week, offering love and support for the wife who had gained 40 pounds in our first 24 months of marriage.

Every morning at Rader, I got up, went for a walk—I didn't want to, but I did it—then I freshened up and went to the dining room for a focused, nutritious breakfast. Table conversation was allowed—encouraged, even—but phone calls were not. The lesson was that other people's emergencies didn't have to disrupt my eating plan. One morning, I received a business call with a commission riding on the conversation. I was determined to take that call, but the nurse told me to put myself first, and let them wait. I conceded. The client waited. And so did the commission.

While at Rader, I learned about portion control, and chewing slowly and purposefully, setting down my fork between bites, and focusing my attention on what I was eating, to give my body a chance to realize I was full and should stop. "There are no taste buds in your throat," they said. "Sip, savor, slow down."

But you see, that wasn't actually the problem. I had learned how to eat politely at my mother's table years before. It wasn't how I ate, so much, as why. And there's really only so much you can do to curb addiction or retrain habits in a week.

I did lose a little weight at Rader, and I did develop some conscious awareness around how much I ate and when and why. And I did go home energized and motivated to eat right, exercise, and lose more weight. I even imagined trying on my wedding dress just to see if it would take me back to my premarital sense of self. But once back home, in my own kitchen, where my familiar routine hung in the air like an old love song, I jumped back into the arms of my old habits. And the weight returned.

I never pulled my wedding dress out of its box, leaving it tucked away with all my illusions of the person I was when it fit. Instead, I sat among framed photos from our special day, studying the vision in each picture and wishing to God I were she. Still.

Sometimes, I overate when I was feeling slimmer, as if it gave me permission to indulge. I also ate when I was feeling fat, as if I'd given up. I overate in times of crisis or grief. Two more years into our marriage, I lost my beloved father. Dad's death, once again, tipped the scales.

My father was killed by a young man he'd hired to work on his home. A boy he believed in, breakfasted with every morning at his kitchen table before they worked, side by side, on home improvements. But once he learned enough about my father's life;

his career, his capacity to pay and the contents of his safe, he came back when he thought the coast was clear, to ransack the house and rob him.

But my parents were home. Confronted by the young man, my father yelled, "Call the police!" to my mother, hiding in the bedroom. As her shaking fingers pressed 911, she heard the gun go off.

For the second time in his life, my father was shot down. But this time, it was absent the hope that comes with the words, "missing in action" a world away from home. This time, he was already home. This time, he'd been gunned down in a much more personal war. And this time, he wasn't coming back.

I couldn't stop eating. Gone was my safe harbor and with it, all the wit and wisdom that had kept me afloat since I was small. I fed my grief with a frenzy, and I knew it. But knowledge is power only if you apply it. And I didn't stand a chance. My grief had carved a hole in my heart, my soul, my stomach, and nothing I ate could fill it. But still, I tried.

I would go into the market and, even before I started gathering groceries, I'd grab some sweet crunchy thing and dig in as I wandered the aisles, trying to think of something to buy that "sounded good." But nothing did, nothing nutritious, anyway. By then I had numbed my appetite for healthy food. At mealtimes, I ate just enough to give me a gateway to dessert.

By now, my handsome husband and I had been married almost five years. I was keenly aware that he'd had a full life before he met me, and I wondered how often he longed for it. I found it a wonder he stuck with me through all of it. But he did.

I didn't want to go on, cramming my life with food, and I didn't want a divorce. But I couldn't see my way out of it. My therapist suggested I move to The Meadows, a treatment center in Arizona that explores the underlying issues of trauma in treating various addictions and disorders, among them, compulsive overeating. Maybe for a month.

I didn't know there was a name for what I was doing. I knew I was overeating, and I knew I couldn't stop, but I didn't understand it as an eating disorder, and I didn't associate it with addiction. I knew I was using food as a painkiller. It had become a habit I couldn't break on my own, supported by my addiction to sugar. I had no idea. It all started, I believe, with my not wanting to go on, and unconsciously choosing a way to redirect my feelings of grief, after my father died. But once I realized my life was going to continue, I knew I didn't want to live this way. This was my motivation for admitting myself to The Meadows.

At The Meadows, hope was an essential part of a program whose steps would lead me to recovery, both emotional and physical. So I packed my bag and moved in. For a month.

Every morning at The Meadows, I woke up in my spare but pleasant room, and spent a few moments remembering where I was and centering my thoughts and expectations for the day. After a guided exercise program, I ate a nutritious breakfast, also monitored, and then met with my counselor to try to get to the core of my compulsive overeating.

In one meeting, the counselor provided a large sheet of paper and a palette of thick, shiny, acrylic paints in rich, vivid colors. My assignment was to paint my eating disorder, to express it, speak to it, get it out, in living color, into the light of day. I had painted be-

fore and was just good enough to feel a little performance anxiety creep in. My counselor assured me that my painting was to be less a work of art and more a work in progress. It was not intended for widespread exhibition; in fact, it was only for me, and the process was as important, more so even, than the product.

That scared me more than anything as I wondered what might come up or out of it. At first, my strokes were gentle, tentative. But the more I addressed the disorder in my mind, the more heated our dialogue, the more I began to slap paint onto the paper, angry that I wasn't getting it, that I couldn't figure out

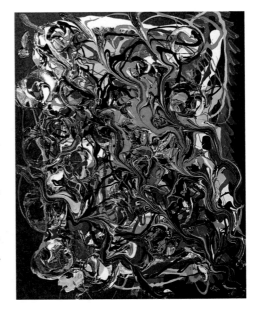

how to resolve my eating disorder on my own. I had heard about people who read books on their eating disorder, and then did what it told them to do, and the problem was resolved. End of story. But not for me. I still felt like I was reading the introduction and had many chapters to go. I couldn't seem to stay on course, to do what they said. I extended my stay at The Meadows another two weeks.

While I didn't feel like I was resolving my eating disorder, I liked living at The Meadows. Other than missing my husband and contact with my children, I felt hopeful, happy, even. As long as I had someone monitoring my every move, I lost weight, and so I felt safe there. Safe from my own behaviors. As long as I remained in the protective custody of their program, I would continue to eat well, lose weight, and feel better about myself. I didn't feel ready to go out into the world, beyond the artificial barriers between myself and my behaviors, to handle my life on my own. Had there been a halfway house, I would have surrendered myself to that.

When I left The Meadows, I was, indeed, slimmer. What scared me about that was how happy I felt, how much better my body looked and felt, and how unsure I was that I would be able to keep up the regimen established for me in such a controlled environment. And I knew exactly what it felt like to backslide into a bowl of ice cream and ride the slippery slope back into obesity. I had been taught what I needed to do to eat nutritious meals and maintain a healthy weight. But I was still missing the part about how to get myself to do it on my own.

You see, it wasn't that I didn't know how to eat right or exercise well. At least I thought I did; my plate was full of seemingly rational weight-loss strategies. What I didn't understand, what I couldn't have known, was that my weight problems stemmed, not only from emotional eating, but also from an addiction to sugar—the raw, artificial, modified, high-fructose, hidden culprit in almost everything I ate. Nobody had talked about that.

Then I discovered the Institute for Integrative Nutrition® (IIN), regarded as the largest nutrition school in the country. I read as much as I could find about the place and felt like it was speaking to me, directly. The instructors talked about learning how to nourish myself in ways other than—in addition to—food. They talked about the staggering numbers of people who wrestle with weight. I started to lift out of my own, insular experience to pay attention to people around me, to hear their stories, and to understand, maybe for the first time, that I was not alone in this. So I enrolled in their program to learn how to nourish myself and, perhaps, others.

Once I found truth in their words at IIN, and value in their program, I decided to learn how to help others. I became a certified health coach.

GOAL

Give a visual, tangible exposure to your emotions and behaviors around eating.

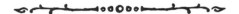

Step One Gather the supplies you will need: a generous piece of construction paper, butcher paper, canvas, linen or newsprint; a set of watercolor or acrylic paints—you can use other mediums, but I prefer the fluid, exploratory, unexpected quality of paint.

Step Two Close your eyes and think about your past and present emotions and behaviors around eating. Picture events and experiences related to eating, not eating, weight, self-esteem or self-loathing, comments or behaviors from others, circumstances, outcomes.

Step Three Let yourself feel the emotions that come up around these behaviors and experiences.

Step Four Open your eyes. Take a moment to look at your blank canvas. Pick up a paint brush and begin to express your emotions, without judgment. Choose as many colors as you wish to depict your wide range of experiences and emotions.

Step Five Explore your painting and the feelings that come up, now.

My own painting, a visual symbol and reminder of my feelings and experiences, appears in this chapter.

Portabella Mushroom Burgers

INGREDIENTS

4 large portabella mushrooms

2 tbsp olive oil

2 avocados

1 Roma tomato, sliced

1 head butter lettuce

1 medium red onion, sliced thick

Salt and pepper to taste

4 slices pepper jack cheese

4 gluten-free hamburger buns

PESTO

¼ cup chopped parsley

¼ almonds

2 cloves garlic, minced

¼ cup balsamic vinegar

½ cup olive oil

1 cup fresh basil

A satisfying alternative to the traditional hamburger

DIRECTIONS

Pesto: In the blender, combine parsley, cilantro, garlic, vinegar, basil, almonds, and oil. Salt and pepper to taste. Blend until combined and refrigerate until ready to use.

Preheat pan or grill. Gently scrub mushroom caps and onions. Drizzle olive oil over each side of mushrooms and onions. When pan or grill is ready, cook mushrooms for 3 to 4 minutes per side. Do the same for the onions.

Meanwhile, mash avocados. Set aside.

In the last minute of cooking, cover mushrooms with Pepper Jack cheese, and grill until cheese has melted. Right before serving, generously top each burger with mashed avocado, pesto, lettuce, tomato and grilled onions.

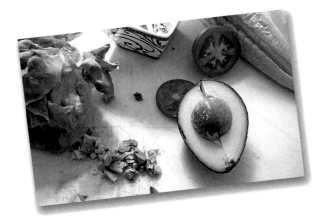

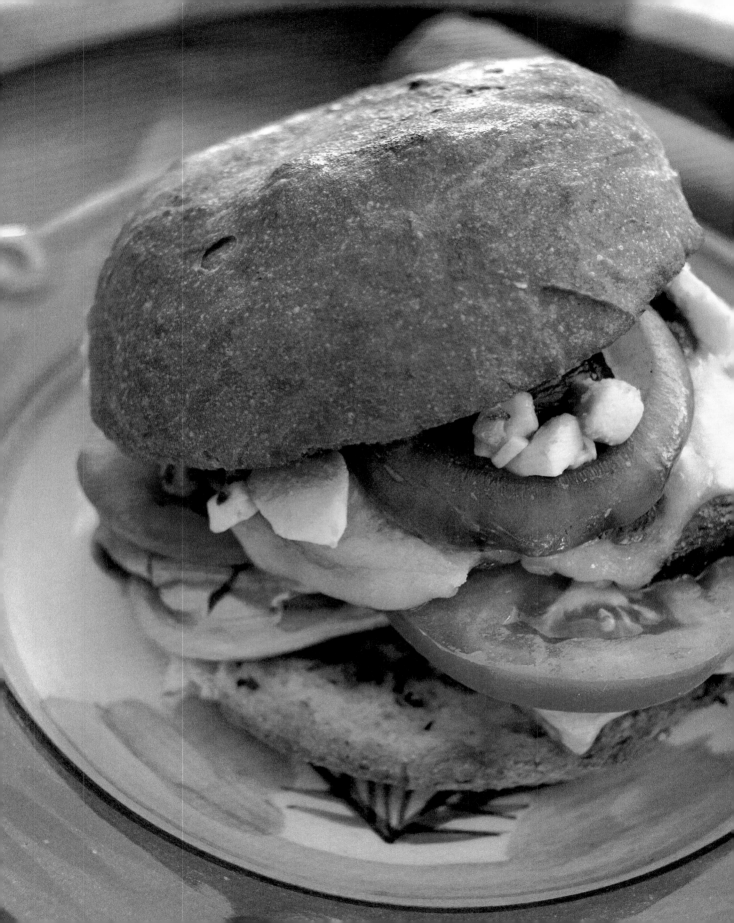

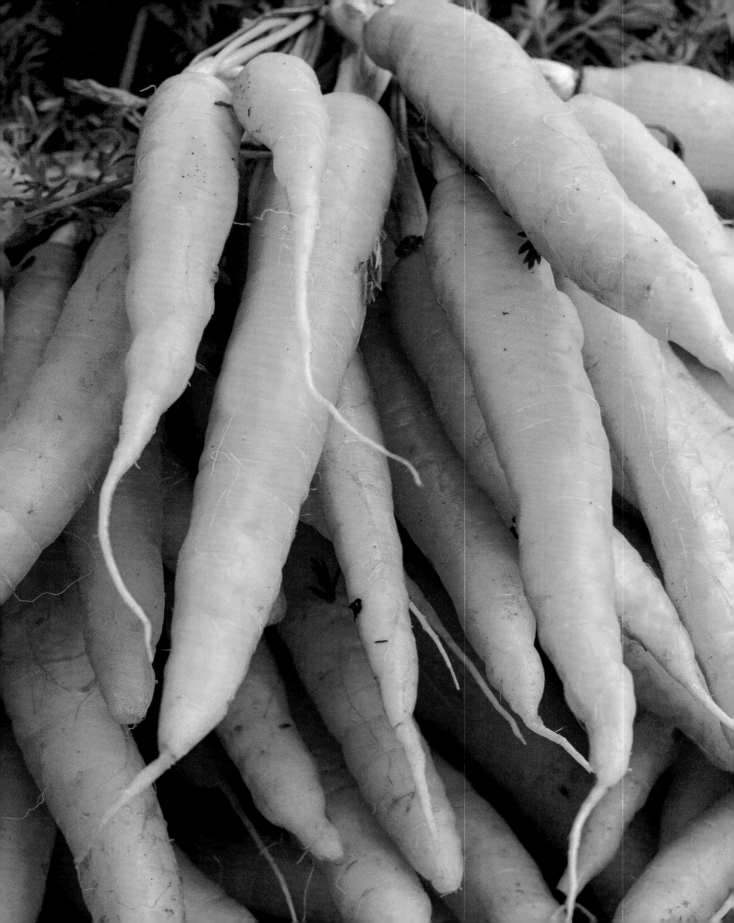

4

Run Harder

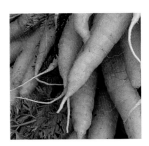

One of the first stories I paid attention to outside my own, which taught me that I am not the only one who has dealt with the effects of living overweight, came from a friend of mine, who recounted her story, over coffee.

Baring your body in front of everyone on a treadmill at the gym is like baring your soul on stage. It takes, pardon the pun, guts. It's not that I believe people must earn the right to wear no more than a skimpy little jog bra and shorts by dieting to the point of extinction—in fact, more power to the people who bare it no matter what—I just have a hard time doing it, myself.

Nevertheless, a friend of mine did. Just that once, when the fans were shut down and the window stuck, when the room got too steamy and, lest she pass out and die, Leslie flung off the tee intended to hide the flab that normally disappears into obscurity beneath black business suits, and pretended to run with abandon in her jog bra and shorts. Just that once.

"Run harder."

The command, from somewhere down the long row of occupied treadmills, broke through Leslie's oxygen-induced trance. She turned her head toward the direction of the voice, as did everyone on every treadmill and, apparently, on every piece of equipment throughout the capacity crowd.

And there, sauntering at a leisurely pace five treadmills down, was Natalie, an 80-year-old woman Leslie knew but hadn't seen for years.

"Excuse me?" Leslie said.

"Run harder."

Leslie had been running, faithfully, obsessively even, for 32 years. Despite the slowing of time, even she thought her 7:30 pace was a pretty decent clip for a day at the gym.

"Why?" She had to ask.

"Because you've gotten fat," Natalie yelled over the roar of the motors. "You're thick. Porky. Run harder."

When Leslie was little, she used to watch a cartoon show on TV called "Shrinking Violet." Every time her feelings got hurt, the character shrank to someone so tiny, viewers could hardly see her any more.

Leslie's face burned somewhere between scarlet and sad. Her eyes stung with tears she hoped no one could see as she turned her head back toward the window where she had been valiantly trying to ignore her reflection. She breathed like a Lamaze student, trying to stall the tears and wishing she could step off the treadmill in the front of her audience and disappear like Violet.

But she couldn't. She still had 45 minutes to go. Besides, she needed the exercise. She *was* porky. Natalie had named it, and Leslie owned it as fast as it came out of Natalie's mouth.

A wonderful thing happens at some point during an energetic run. A sense of well-being takes over. Leslie, actually, for the moment, let it go.

But Natalie didn't. Having finished her stroll, she wandered up behind Leslie, slapped her on the shoulder and said, "You have gained weight, haven't you. You're porky. You're going to have to run harder." And she continued on out through the door.

The flame returned to Leslie's cheeks as fresh tears spilled onto the treadmill. She still had 10 minutes to go.

Usually, after her run, Leslie slips into a Speedo swimsuit and stretches out her muscles with some laps in the outdoor pool. She stepped off the treadmill and looked out the window at the glistening water that normally seduces her. Yet suddenly she had no idea how to stuff herself into a swimsuit, in public.

Just before she left the gym, she noticed a black telephone sitting on a small desk in the corner. She picked up the receiver on the old-school phone and dialed the cell number of a girlfriend. Just hearing her friend's voice was like a balm as she answered the phone, and Leslie poured out her story with all the tears she had stemmed on the treadmill.

Her friend's anger at Natalie's comments hit Leslie like something between a hug and a high five. She ordered Leslie into the pool.

Nearly an hour later, after Leslie had finished her swim and her shower, the door to the locker room swung open. In walked her best friend, who had left her desk and made the drive over to the gym.

"I am here," she said, "to help you get back into your day. I am here to congratulate you for exercising every single day of the week. I am here to remind you what's important and what's not. And I am here to take you to lunch."

That night, Leslie decided to offer Natalie the chance to grow. She found her e-mail address and sat down to send her a letter:

Dear Natalie:

When I was in fifth grade, the church choir director offered us a special treat at the end of rehearsal: a piece of solid milk chocolate wrapped in foil to resemble a ladybug. As he made his way among fifty 10-year-olds seated along three risers, he held out a cardboard box in front of child after child, each of whom reached into the box and selected a piece of chocolate.

Halfway down the front row, he extended the box to my sister, a little slip of a thing who quickly picked out her ladybug. As he stepped in front of me, I reached my hand toward him in eager anticipation of my chocolate. But he withdrew the box.

Perhaps, in response to the horror registering across my face, he returned the box to my reach and said, "I guess you can have one. I guess you're just what we call pleasingly plump."

My sister returned her chocolate to the box, took my hand, and got me out of there.

Natalie, you have no idea who you were talking to today, no idea what you did to my self-esteem with your unkind words. I tell you this story not to ruin your day but in hopes that should you ever feel the inclination to hurl your criticism across the gym again, you will refrain.

And may I remind you that anyone who has ever gained weight is already painfully aware of it.

Leslie studied her words, already sensing the satisfaction in having spoken up for herself. Yet she realized it didn't matter whether her words inspired Natalie or if she ever received a response. She smiled and hit "send."

Leslie still goes to the gym, still runs on the treadmill, still swim laps in the pool, still curses the 10 pounds sitting between her and "perfection," still loves chocolate, still remembers what's most important and what's not. . . and where she fits into that.

You see, it isn't about "running harder." It's time to forgive ourselves and others, and let the weight of insult go.

All the bullying and name calling we endured as children—or adults—returns to us long after the others stop their banter. As it persists in our mind, we are doing the same thing to ourselves. And it is even worse until we get the tools to understand why we keep the torment alive and present.

Emotional recovery starts when we can stop beating ourselves up. Once we realize our value is infinite and indivisible; we are worthy, we are enough, and we have every right to take our place and make our own imprint on this earth. Our lives have value simply because we are alive. We tend to know this about everyone else; it is time to believe it of ourselves.

GOAL

Create the benevolent armor known as self esteem to guard and protect yourself from potential wounding inflicted by the "imposing influence" or thoughtless and unkind words of others.

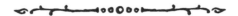

PART ONE

Step One   Review the chart on "12 Steps to Better Health" on the next page, and listed below. Notice how many steps are missing from your daily path and which ones you might want to introduce as part of the self care that will help forge your self esteem.

1. Drink more water
2. Practice cooking
3. Experiment with whole grains
4. Increase sweet vegetables
5. Increase leafy green vegetables
6. Experiment with protein
7. Eat fewer processed foods
8. Make a habit of nurturing your body
9. Have healthy relationships
10. Enjoy regular physical activity
11. Find work you love
12. Develop a spiritual practice

In Leslie's story, "Run Harder," she had chosen healthy relationships she could call on to receive loving support, validation of who she is and her inherent worth, and recognition of her accomplishments. Leslie nurtured her body by exercising

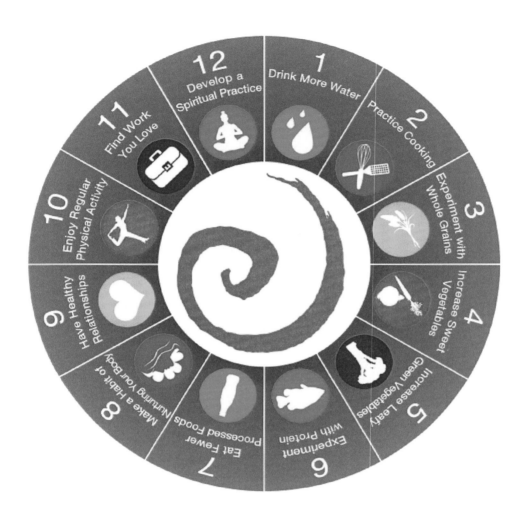

1. Drink More Water
2. Practice Cooking
3. Experiment with Whole Grains
4. Increase Sweet Vegetables
5. Increase Leafy Green Vegetables
6. Experiment with Protein
7. Eat Fewer Processed Foods
8. Make a Habit of Nurturing Your Body
9. Have Healthy Relationships
10. Enjoy Regular Physical Activity
11. Find Work You Love
12. Develop a Spiritual Practice

and fueled it by going to lunch afterward. If you don't have a trusted friend or family member readily available when the clouds come in, engage your own spiritual practice to help get you through the storm. You can do it. You're worth it.

PART TWO

Step One   Let yourself feel your feelings. Sit with them, experience them. Then express them, get them out and into words.

Step Two   Pore through a magazine or other series of images, online. Focus on a certain photograph or other visual representation. Study it, describe it, consider why you chose it and notice how you feel.

Step Three   Give yourself 60 seconds to write a poem. No edits. No tweaks. Just write and see what comes up. Pay attention to how you feel as you write your poem and as you read it to yourself. Think about what your chosen image stirred in you.

Mushroom Lettuce Wraps

WRAP INGREDIENTS

1 lb baby bell mushrooms

½ cup diced onion

1 14.5-oz can diced tomatoes

2 chipotle peppers

2 tbsp avocado oil

Salt and pepper to taste

RICE INGREDIENTS

2 cups brown rice

4 cups chicken stock (organic Better
    than Bouillon chicken base)

½ cup diced onion

1 14.5-oz can diced tomatoes

2 tbsp coconut oil

Salt and pepper to taste

A light, vegetarian version of the traditional taco

DIRECTIONS

Heat oil in sauté pan. Once pan is hot, add onion and cook for about 3 minutes, then add mushrooms and cook for 5 more minutes. Puree tomato and chipotle peppers, and add to mushroom mixture. Season to taste. Cook for 10 more minutes. Remove from heat. Serve over butter lettuce or romaine.

EXTRAS

guacamole or avocado • caramelized onions • beans

Spanish Rice

DIRECTIONS

Heat a medium saucepan and add oil. Brown rice and onion. Sauté for about 7 minutes, stirring constantly, then add the tomatoes and chicken stock. Once it comes to a boil, reduce heat to medium low, and cook for 35 to 40 minutes until all liquid is absorbed. Remove from heat.

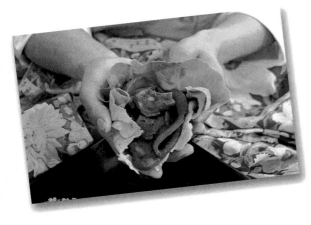

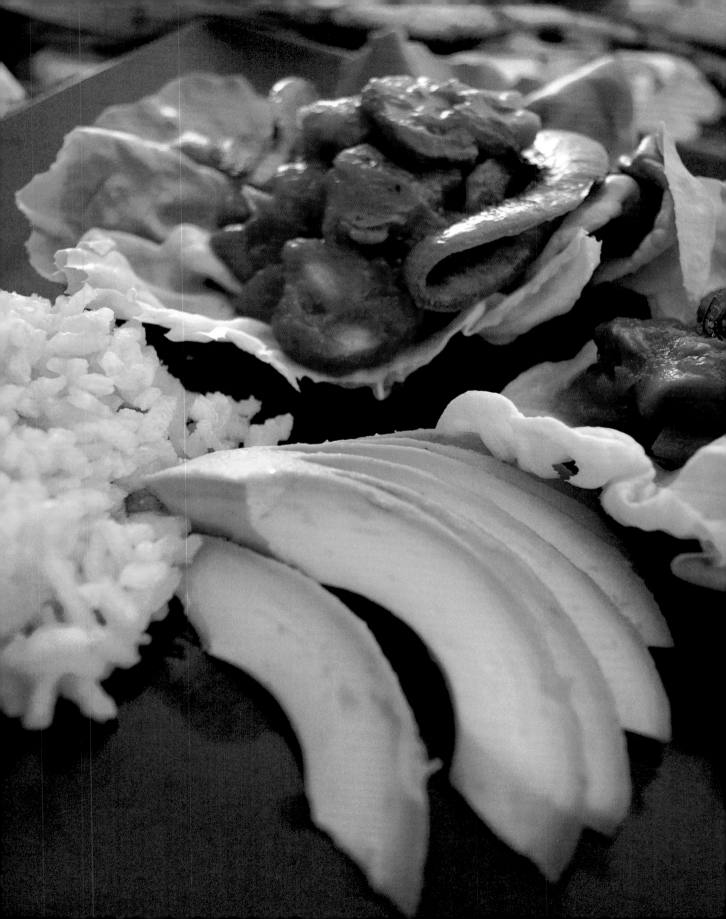

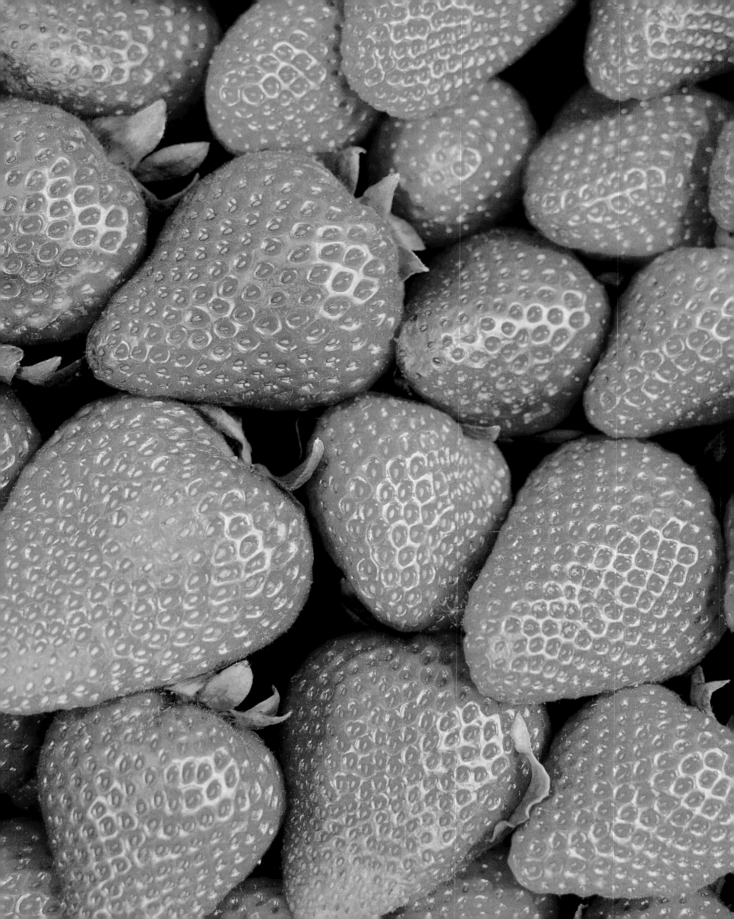

5

Happiest Place on Earth

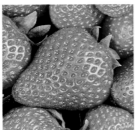

It's supposed to be the happiest place on earth. And actually, she was just as excited as her young daughter to go to Disneyland. Upon arrival, when her child flung wide her arms and spun round and round, saying, "We're here; we're finally here," she felt the same way.

My friend, Carolyn, had waited a long time for this family adventure. She had waited until she had the funds. She had waited until her child was old enough to enjoy it. She had *intended* to wait until she had lost her baby weight, so she, too, could have fun. Yet instead, she had actually gained weight and was packing an extra 100 pounds on this trip.

"My daughter weighed 6 pounds at birth," says Carolyn. "But I had gained 106, myself. That's just not good math. Nobody talked to me about weight during my pregnancy; they were just so happy about my child. Afterward, that's all they talked about. And when the postpartum depression set in, I lost the ability to deal with it. Depression led to disappointment, which led to disgust. Once I reached 250 pounds, I refused to look in the mirror."

Within the first hour of wandering around Disneyland with her family, Carolyn's ankles gave out. From heat, from weight, from despair. She simply couldn't stand it. Her husband quietly rented a wheelchair, and she took her place among the elderly and infirm parked outside each attraction.

As she sat outside "Mickey's Toontown," wondering how she had gotten to this place in her life and waiting for her child to exit the fun house, Carolyn felt a caress across her back. She turned in her chair to see the Goofy character, his head cocked to the side in a sad tilt. "When you get a pity pat from a cartoon character," she says, "it's time to do something about your situation."

Carolyn had never been fat before. In fact, growing up, it wasn't allowed. Not in her family and, pretty much, not in her town. Her parents weighed themselves every morning and asked the same of her. Maintaining weight was a function of discipline and a sign of respect. For herself and her family. Carolyn was always grateful that, although she had been born with broad shoulders, she had always been thin.

Until the baby. And the divorce. And all the other pressures that came along the way.

"I was in a state of being my parents couldn't comprehend," says Carolyn. "I became anxious whenever they came to visit, knowing they would be disappointed in me. My mother would tear up and say, "Ah, Carolyn,' in her Lauren Bacall voice. My father simply wouldn't make eye contact with me. I've always been a daddy's girl and have spent my life trying to please him by being more like my mother. It was something I just couldn't deliver."

The day Carolyn decided to lose weight was the day she looked at her little girl and decided to reclaim her life, so she could be here for hers. She actually looked into something called bariatric surgery. Essentially, weight loss would be achieved by reducing the size of the stomach or by re-routing the small intestines to a small stomach pouch.

"I saw bariatric surgery as a quick fix," says Carolyn, "which was appealing to the desperate side of me. I didn't have faith I could harness my out-of-control eating on my own. But I also wondered if it would be a temporary solution. Once the doctor laid out the process in front of me, I realized it wasn't a quick fix, and I thought maybe I could put that kind of effort into a healthier lifestyle."

Still, she knew she couldn't do it alone. She joined Weight Watchers, where she found people larger and smaller than she. She found people who would cheer her on, people with a sense of humor.

"I had developed my own sense of humor," she says, "as a way to connect with people since I couldn't count on my looks. My family didn't have a sense of humor. To them, I was the elephant in the room. At Weight Watchers, we were all elephants in the room."

Carolyn knew she needed to combine exercise with her new eating habits, but she didn't have the strength or stamina to do much. She started by sitting in a chair and doing arm circles in front of the TV. Then she lifted her foot off the floor and drew the letters of the alphabet in the air. It was a start.

Getting fit is a gift to myself

Eventually, she added walking to her routine and, finally, she braved the sea of spandex and set foot in a gym where she was delighted to find members of all sizes and shapes. For the next 18 months, she made it a habit, every day, like brushing her teeth, as she worked through weight machines and took a walk on the treadmill. By the end of her weight-loss journey, Carolyn had lost 120 pounds. And, five years hence, she has maintained her workout schedule and her weight loss.

"At first I was so disappointed in my body," she says. "But then I realized my body didn't betray me; I betrayed it. My body was more than happy to oblige whatever I asked of it, particularly once I started taking care of it. I had to work my tush off to get there, but I was finally working with my body instead of against it. I stopped telling myself I needed to lose weight and started saying I needed to get in better shape.

"Losing weight sounded like losing a part of myself, which scared me. Getting fit is a gift to myself that takes nothing away from me but instead, gave me back my life."

Five years after Carolyn lost more than 100 pounds, she returned with her teenage daughter to Disneyland. Together they mastered "The Matterhorn," got drenched on "Splash Mountain," sang their way around the globe in "It's a Small World," and tucked quite nicely into "Mickey's Toontown."

The place to begin emotional and physical recovery from living overweight is intolerance. You are no longer willing to feel bad, either physically or emotionally. You are no longer willing to subject yourself to the opinions or observations of others. You are no longer willing to suffer the ill effects of excess weight or obesity, such as heart disease, diabetes, arthritis. You can no longer tolerate a lifestyle that keeps you from your inherent joy and the engaged, productive life you deserve.

Goal

Identify your need for emotional recovery from living with weight issues.

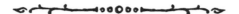

Step One   Write down a brief story of an experience you have had that illustrates your connection to each of the emotional states listed below:

- Low self-esteem
- Dissatisfaction with body image
- Feelings of being a failure
- Feeling like you are on the outside looking in
- Feeling like no one knows the real you

Step Two   Read through each story to get an understanding of the feelings generated by the experience.

Step Three   Think about the same feelings that come up for you around your weight issues, as you draw parallels to the stories.

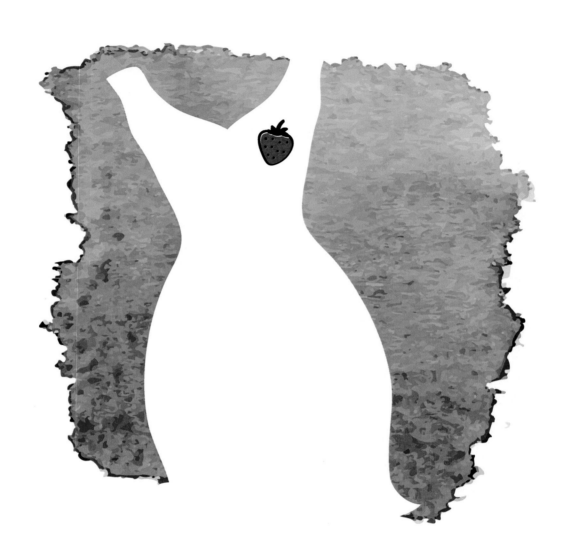

BBQ Pineapple Pulled Pork Pizza

GLUTEN-FREE PIZZA CRUST INGREDIENTS

- 2 ½ cups almond flour
- 1 ½ cup arrowroot
- 2 tbsp olive oil
- 2 tsp baking powder
- 1 tsp garlic powder
- 1 tbsp Italian seasoning
- 2 tsp salt
- ½ tsp black pepper
- ⅔ cup coconut milk
- 4 eggs

BBQ PULLED PORK INGREDIENTS

- 1 lb boneless pork shoulder or pork loin
- ¼ tsp freshly ground black pepper
- ¼ tsp salt
- ½ cup water
- ½ cup barbecue sauce
- 2 cups Mozzarella
- 1 ½ cups pineapple chunks

Tangy, gluten-free Hawaiian-style flatbread

DIRECTIONS

Preheat oven to 425 degrees.

Crust: Grease round pizza pan or rimmed cookie sheet with coconut oil. Mix all dry ingredients in medium bowl until well combined, and set aside. In a separate small bowl, whip eggs with coconut milk and oil; then add the wet mixture to the dry, and mix until well incorporated. The batter will be quite runny. Spread batter onto greased pizza pan, and bake for 10 minutes. Remove from oven and set aside.

Pork: Rinse pork shoulder and pat dry. Rub salt and pepper over pork, and place in slow cooker. Add water. Cook on low setting for 6 hours, until pork is very tender. Remove pork from slow cooker and discard remaining liquid. Using two forks, shred pork. Add BBQ sauce and mix well.

Pizza: Top pizza bread with Mozzarella, shredded pork and pineapple chunks. Bake at 425 for 10 minutes or until cheese is melted.

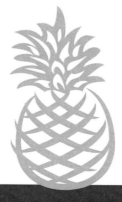

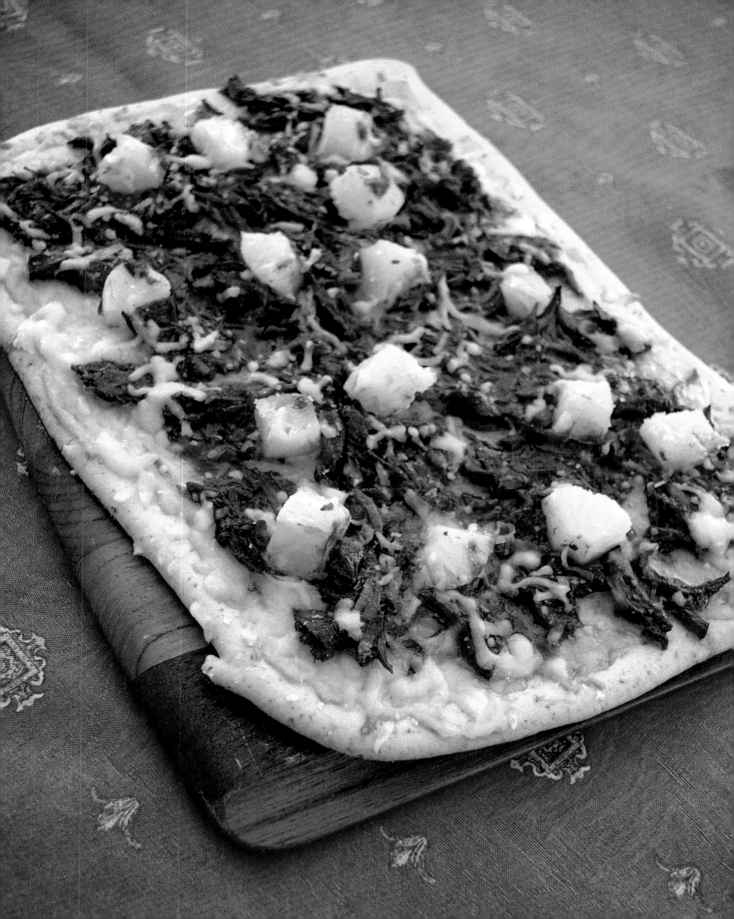

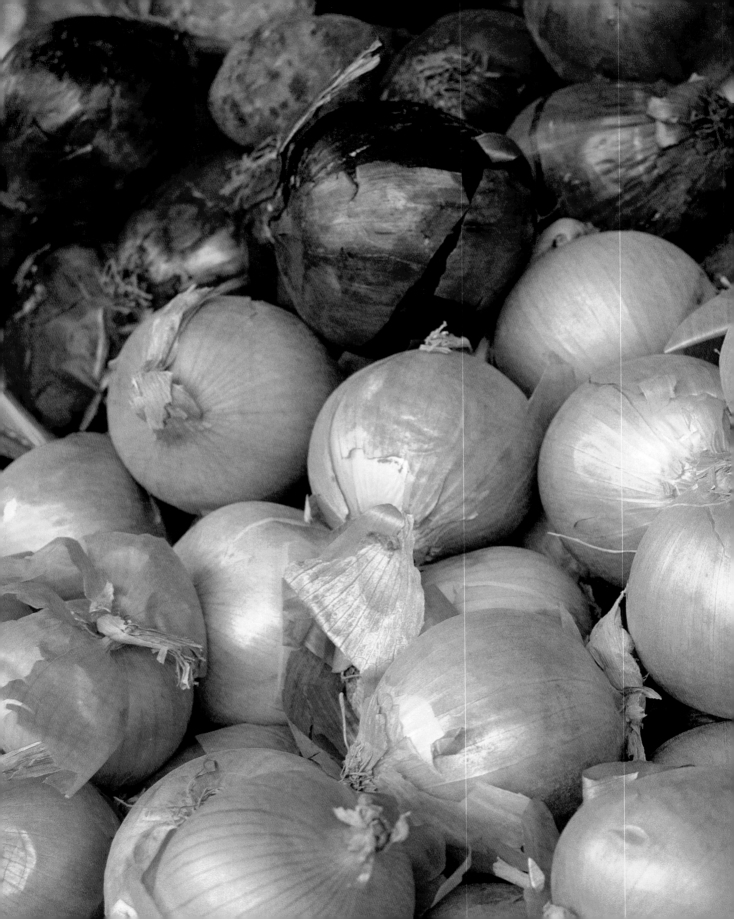

6

State of Grace

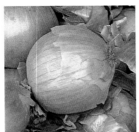 My own path toward emotional and physical recovery from living overweight has had forks in the road (pun intended), some of which led me off track, and others that brought me even closer to my wellness destination. One of those has been my spiritual path.

Back in 1973, a decade before I met my current husband, I left Washington, DC and flew to Houston as a newly separated woman, facing divorce. I did not know anyone in Texas except my sister, waiting to offer me, my two children and our dog a soft landing. My sister had an apartment in Houston, filled with her things, but she invited us to make ourselves at home, and even offered to send for our household goods. Where she planned to put it all was less important than giving us a sense of security, of belonging, of peace.

Two months later we were evicted, not having known that the management didn't allow pets or children. The first few places I tried to rent shunned me as a single or divorced mother, saying they didn't rent to "my kind." It was another era. Desperate, I drove to nearby churches, seeking shelter and the suggestion of a more permanent solution. Again, the word "divorce" tripped me at the door.

I had never been on my own before. A 30-year-old woman with two children and a dog is hardly alone, but I felt completely isolated from the embrace of society. At the time, I had not yet completed my college education, so I came across as unskilled and unemployable. I got the message that a college education could be a golden key to productivity and prosperity. In the meantime, I needed a job.

I took the only position I was offered, a sales job on straight commission. It may sound close to insanity for a young mother with so much responsibility to take a job with no guarantees. But it served to motivate me, and I fought my way to record-breaking sales.

Those of us given to emotional eating tend to gain or lose weight during times of stress. I believed at the time, and I know for sure, now, this was actually one of the most difficult and trying periods of my life. It also was when I realized I could gain weight while eating very little. I was too stressed, too busy, trying too hard to take time to eat right. I ate on the go, grabbing whatever was within reach. It wasn't much, and it wasn't expensive, but it was usually laced or loaded with sugar, and held together by hydrogenated fats. And so, I gained weight. Again.

Getting fat at a time when I was trying to get a job and, once I had the job, trying to present myself and my products professionally, was like inviting Cinderella to the ball without the benefits of a fairy godmother. I had the goods, I could excel in my job, but I didn't look like it. And I certainly didn't feel like it. I imagined others wouldn't be able to see my potential either, through all the layers of self-doubt.

My life was off balance, out of whack. It would be years before I understood that there is more to nourishing myself than eating nutritious food. Through the Institute of Integrative Nutrition®, I learned about "primary foods™," the nurturing aspects of life— relationships, spirituality, career, finance, creativity, physical exercise—that also had to be healthy in my life before I could begin to find balance or even hope to steady the scales.

Whether or not I ate and what I put in my mouth seemed like the only things I could govern. But even that slipped out of my grasp. When a co-worker told me he'd noticed I was gaining weight, his comment landed like condemnation.

I had gotten my job through a placement agency, which would rake in 25% of my commissions for the first three months on the job. Trouble was, although I had laid the foundation to build the kind of trust and relationships that should lead to sales, I hadn't as of yet, closed a sale. My boss gave me an ultimatum: Make a sale within the next 10 days, or I'd be fired. I plied my panic with chocolate and cheese, consuming my fear and disappointment until I was fed up but not full.

And then the phone rang. On the ninth day, one of my carefully cultivated clients made a sizeable purchase. I put down my fork and picked up a pen. It was a start.

During that time of transition, someone told me about the Unity Church, a spiritual/ philosophical movement best known to many through its *Daily Word* devotional publication. I actually had read the *Daily Word* to my grandmother every morning as a young adult, and I remember feeling uplifted by its message. And I was with my grandmother when, as a little girl, I attended a church revival in Pasadena, CA, led by the Filmores, founders of the Unity movement, which later became a church.

I started attending Sunday services at the Unity Church in Houston. It was the only place, besides my office and the grocery store, I felt comfortable going without an escort. Again, another era. What I found there was hope, healing and a whole new community. I felt safe. I had a sense of place, not only at church on Sundays but at holiday tables and other events. I belonged.

The messages I received through Unity Church taught me to believe in myself. I learned where my essential energy comes from, which can help me withstand temptation. The parables I heard from the pulpit shared by Reverend John D. Rankin and Reverend Howard Caesar on Sundays reached me in real ways. While spirituality and faith show up differently for different people, I learned there is a God who lives within us, and all we have to do is ask for the strength and the direction, and we will be guided. It took me a long time to learn this, but I finally did, as I came out of a negative mindset and into a place of peace and acceptance.

hope, healing, and a whole new community

In those early days with the Unity Church, whenever I would meditate, it would make my world small enough that I could find peace within it. That still, small voice would say, "Come to me, my child." Whenever I asked God for guidance on the next right thing, He never actually told me, but He let me know He would watch over me. Sometimes I made the right choice, and sometimes I didn't. But I still had Him there, to guide me.

A friend of mine told me she would know I was OK once I was able to turn my attention away from my troubles and toward others in need. Once I felt safe and secure, I realized I never wanted another woman to go through what I had. I wanted to share with others my faith that they would never truly be alone as long as they reached for the hand of God. He who lives within us and around us—all we have to do is ask Him for help or strength or direction or comfort, and trust it shall be so. I believed that.

I wanted women to know they are neither bad nor wrong for the difficult decisions they must make. I wanted women to trust in their own wisdom and resources, secure in the knowledge that both are divinely given. I learned to love the saying, "I made the best decision I could with the tools I had at the time, and with new tools and new information, I will make a new decision."

I became so involved in my church and my support of women in transition, I started to hear suggestions from my community that I should consider pastoring or politics. Confident that politics was not my platform, I began to consider ministerial school.

I had remarried—this time, for good—and I was actually in a perfect position to go back to school. But, so was my husband, Nic. In 2000, at age 57, he began medical school to become a doctor of osteopathy. So, I started slowly. I invited Nic to a couples' workshop at Unity Village in Missouri.

Following a deeply inspiring weekend for us both, I stayed on for two more weeks of additional coursework. And I knew, probably by the end of that first weekend, but definitely upon successful completion of my coursework, that I was destined to be ordained.

As a child, I had never done well in school. Somewhere, deep inside, I believed I was smart, but nothing in my marks or my mother's remarks confirmed that. All these years later, a friend in Michigan encouraged me to continue taking classes and to apply for work-experience credit. She saw something in me I was not able to see in myself. After a battery of tests I learned, for the first time at almost 60, that I have dyslexia, a learning disorder characterized by difficult reading. What that taught me is that I am completely capable of learning, just a little bit differently.

I continued my adjunct coursework until my husband graduated from medical school in 2004. That year, I applied to Unity School and was accepted for the spring semester 2005. Concurrently during my coursework at Unity, I applied to Ottawa University in Kansas City, a faith-based, student-centered university with a flexible curriculum to enable a diversity of students to "prepare for a lifetime of significance." Something I'd been seeking for 60 years. I was ordained into the Unity Church in 2007 and, one year later, I graduated from Ottawa University with honors.

The process of becoming ordained taught me some very important things about myself and my God, about infinite worth, and that all things are possible. The more I read about how Jesus sought to show others how to realize their divine potential, the more I realized I was not nearly as interested in what ordination could do for me as I was in what I could do for other women who found themselves in similar situations to mine when I first came to Houston.

As an ordained minister, I wanted to create a space where women and also men knew they were welcomed, cared for, listened to, included and honored for their skills and talents. I wanted them to know there is a God who lives within them, a loving God, who has our best interests at heart. I wanted to encourage people to quiet their racing minds and slow their pounding hearts just enough to hear that "still, small voice" of reassurance.

I wanted to help people understand that the hole left in their hearts after a divorce or other significant loss can be filled by the Spirit instead of food or other addictive substances. In this space, I wanted to encourage people to walk with their shoulders squared and heads held high, knowing that no matter what had happened in their past, they had a spiritual home where they would be welcomed, loved, appreciated and included.

During the week, I was working with my husband in his medical practice, and during the weekends, I was doing my work at church. Burning the candle at both ends, I began to flame out. I knew I needed to make a decision. In working with my husband to educate his patients on the effects of their nutrition on their bodies, I truly was doing God's work, by helping men and women learn to make healthy food choices to nourish their bodies and their lives. Spirituality is one of the key elements among primary foods™.

Years later, my passion for helping people, particularly women in need, is still within me. I find I am able to combine spirituality, hypnotherapy and health coaching to address most issues women are facing, today. Myself included.

My hope for others is that you, too, will find your passionate pursuit, trusting that you have what it takes to get there. For I have proved in my life that my friend was right. Once we can lift our sights up and out of our own inner struggles, shifting our gaze toward the needs of others, we begin to move into our life's balance, spiritually, emotionally, and physically. And our weight becomes secondary.

Goal

Clarify and manifest the life you want.

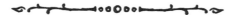

When my neighbor was 3 years old, she would run into her preschool every morning, fling her arms in the air, and announce, "I'm back!"—so filled was she with excitement for herself and the day ahead. We can all greet the day that way once we discover our life's passionate pursuits.

This is an exercise to help your subconscious mind lead you to your heart's desire. Take some time with this because you deserve it.

Step One   Turn off your phone. Light a candle. Close your eyes, and breathe. Slowly, deeply, evenly. Center your focus on your *self*.

Step Two   Think about what you want for your life in the next five years. When you are ready, open your eyes, seeing yourself as you might be five years down the road. Using as much detail as possible, describe, in writing, your home— your living room, bedroom, kitchen, your wardrobe, your car, your *self*.

Consider color, texture, shape, size, style. How do you dress? What do you eat for breakfast? With whom do you share your morning? Do you exercise? Read the paper, check your iPad, walk the dog, or rush out the door to your office, classroom, studio, salon?

How does your day proceed? How do you spend your time, and with whom? What is your passionate pursuit? Do you come home to make dinner, meet friends or colleagues for cocktails, head to the gym, the restaurant, the market? What becomes of your evening?

Step Three   Now put your writing away for safekeeping, and let your subconscious mind go to work on creating your vision. Here is what became of mine:

I was single and just beginning to develop my career when I described my vision of the passionate pursuits of my life. I envisioned a spacious home with a balcony off the master bedroom. I saw my business attire lined up like suitors in my closet, well heeled with shoes toeing the line. I saw myself sitting on boards of directors and joining prestigious business affiliations. I read articles published about my financial finesse and community contributions. And I let myself experience it in my mind as if it were really happening.

Within a few years, I had moved from my rented townhome and was standing on the balcony outside the master bedroom of my new home, when I realized my list had come true with the exception of the man of my dreams with whom to share my life. Even he showed up, just a few years later. My subconscious mind had continued to work on my heart's desires until I met my husband of now 27 years. You really can direct your intentions, but you have to get clear about what they really are, first.

Oatmeal Chocolate-Chip Cookies

INGREDIENTS

½ cup almond flour

1 cup rolled oats

½ tsp baking soda

½ tsp baking powder

½ tsp salt

1 tbsp coconut flour

½ cup coconut sugar

1 cup chocolate chips

2 eggs

¼ cup coconut oil

2 tbsp honey

2 tsp vanilla extract

The perfect pairing of indulgent chocolate and health-boosting oats

DIRECTIONS

Preheat oven to 350 degrees.

In a large bowl, combine all dry ingredients, including chocolate chips, and set aside.

In a small saucepan, melt coconut oil. Then remove from heat and add vanilla and honey.

In a medium bowl, beat eggs, and add oil mixture; mix well. Next, add wet ingredients to dry and, with a rubber spatula, mix until well incorporated.

Place golf ball-sized balls of dough on a cookie sheet lined with parchment or a silicone baking sheet. Bake for 14 to 17 minutes, until slightly golden around the edges.

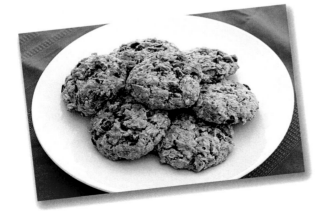

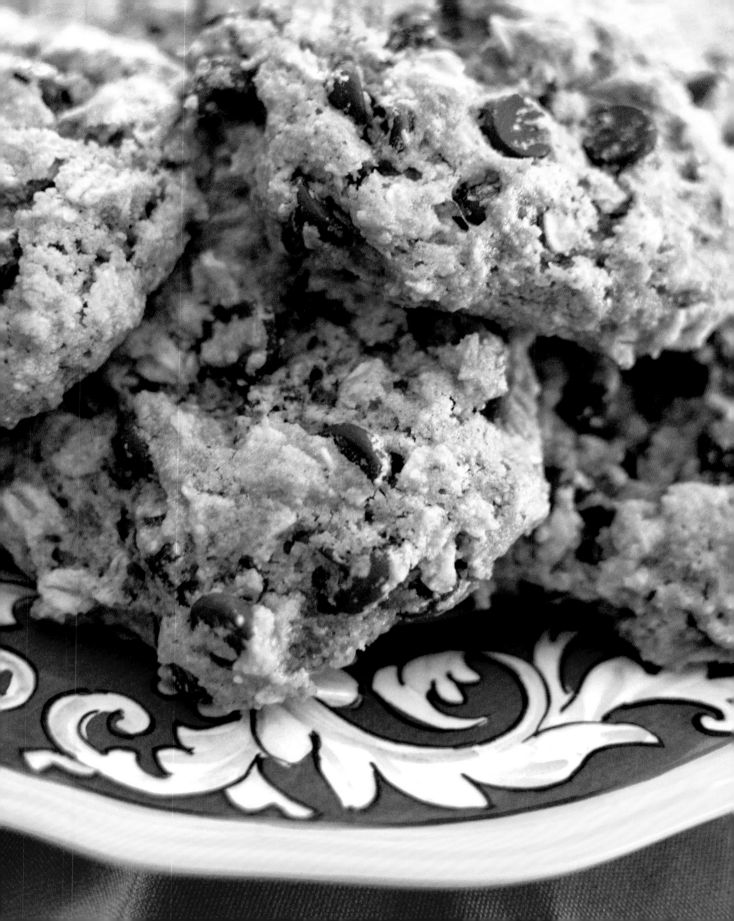

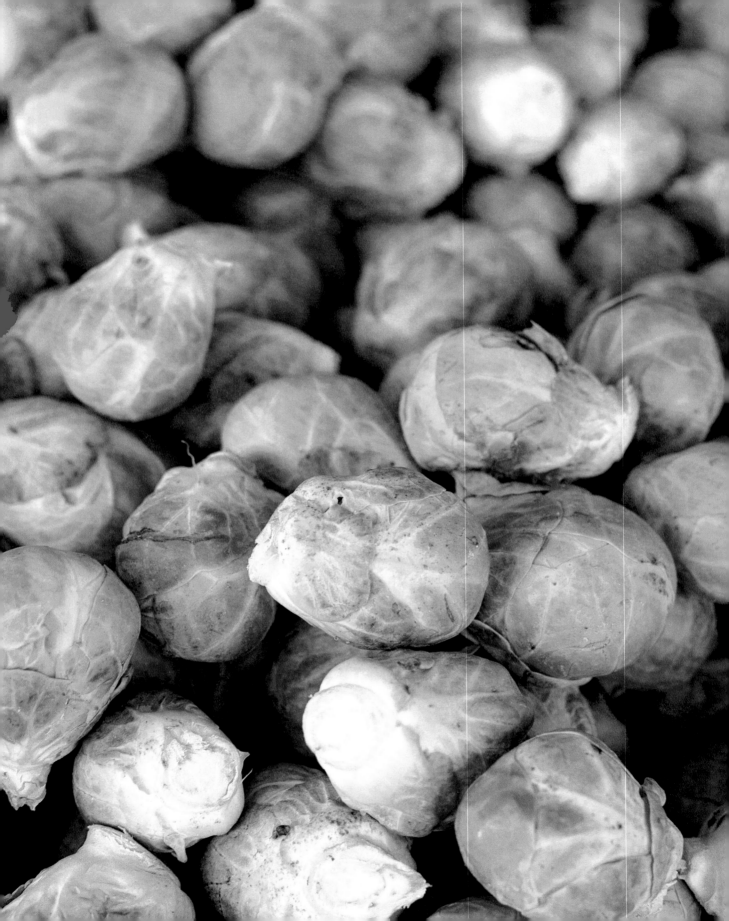

7

When It's Not About Food

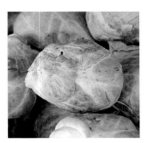 By all appearances, I had the traditional trappings of a happy life—intelligence, career success, travel, beautiful children, happy home, and marriage to a handsome doctor. But I also still harbored a secret frustration I had not been able to solve. My weight. Whether it was too high or too low or even just right, it consumed my thoughts, my actions, my joy.

I had devoured books, turned dieting into a lifestyle and, actually, everything had worked. For a while. As armed as I was with information and experience, I still didn't know how to create a healthy lifestyle I could sustain. Until I learned about the Institute for Integrative Nutrition® (IIN), which trains health coaches to "educate and support people to build healthy new habits and create sustainable lifestyle changes."

As I looked into the school, its history and its mission, I realized the best way to solve my issues was to learn enough from IIN to understand how to teach others to do the same. After considerable time, training, thought and reflection, I am finally able to come from a place of knowing and understanding as I escort clients along our journeys to recovery.

Through my IIN coursework, I studied the basic science and nutrition that relates to the consumption and digestion of food. What food is made of, and how it is broken down in the body and converted to basic building blocks for our growth and mainte-nance. I learned which food types, like sugar, are harmful, and which are beneficial, like antioxidants, protein, fats, and carbohydrates.

I also studied more than 100 different types of food plans and theories currently discussed in the media. Experts in the field explained the relative merits and problems with each, concluding that no single plan is right for everyone. Bioindividuality™, the degree of variation in life, is what sets us all apart. Perhaps most importantly, I learned why I had experienced such difficulty with and guilt over my own weight and how little it had to do with food. I also learned what I could do about it while helping others.

During a coaching session, one of my clients revealed she had a very hard time eating alone, in public. Through a guided visualization, she explored her physical and emotional responses to the idea of entering a restaurant on her own, taking her seat at an empty table, and lingering during the waiting periods between ordering and eating. She felt the heat of embarrassment flush her face. She said she felt exposed, lonely, self-conscious.

I invited my client to think about a time during her childhood, when she experienced, not necessarily for the same reason, the same feelings.

She thought back to an episode, when she was 6 years old, in a doctor's office, where the nurse was trying, unsuccessfully, to draw a blood sample. After six, maybe more sticks with the needle, my client, feeling the discomfort, the fear, the loneliness and her embarrassment at the tears that began to course down her cheeks, hid her face beneath her corduroy coat.

I asked her where she got the idea that crying was an inappropriate response to her ordeal. She explained the standards of decorum her mother had set for the family. We now had a place from which to work on her emotions around eating alone in public.

Sometimes, in our coaching sessions, we talk about meal planning and menus, recipes and the kinds of fresh food that can be found at a farmers market. Because sometimes, our focus is on learning how to feed ourselves; literally, what to make for dinner that will satisfy and nourish the family. Other times, we look at the emotional issues driving what we eat, when we eat and why. Food is, quite often, not the reason we overeat. It is the coping tool that causes the weight gain, but it is rarely the source of the problem. In that case, we look into what is going on in our lives, our hearts, our minds, often well before we ever come to the dinner table.

Today, in partnership with my husband, Clarence L. Nicodemus, DO, PhD (a fully licensed physician in Neuromusculoskeletal Medicine) as well as Chef Paola Mikes, and a team of certified health coaches, I work through our company, Advanced Osteopathy, a medical practice that addresses physical pain, paired with a program of preventive medicine counseling, and health coaching. Together we have formed a comprehensive mind-and-body healing center for our clients.

Using a gentle, non-invasive technique, Dr. Nicodemus helps the body understand it can heal itself under the right conditions. People want to know that any program they participate in for their health is honest and based on medical science. As part of my health coaching, Dr. Nicodemus reviews each client's medical history, and looks for conditions that may need attention as the person explores dietary changes. Pre-existing conditions, such as hypertension and diabetes, are excellent reasons one should consider a carefully developed food plan. Dr. Nicodemus is available to explain the physiological and biochemical underpinnings of the digestive process and to explain how certain foods are especially beneficial for a specific condition.

Understanding that emotional and physical issues can affect the well-being of the body, I work from an insightful, non-judgmental, empathic approach to resolution. Chef Mikes teaches how to use fresh, organic, nutrient-packed ingredients to cook nutritious meals. Through health coaching, we also present workshops, seminars, and group and individual sessions designed to help participants discover healthier food and lifestyle choices to foster a more vibrant life.

Goal

We want to ferret out the experiences in our lives that have ignited lingering emotions, which surface in other, more current contexts, and motivate us to seek solace in or sometimes rejection of food or the circumstances around eating.

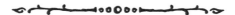

Step One Sit down in a place that feels safe, and make yourself comfortable. Close your eyes, and take in a few deep breaths, inhaling through your nose and exhaling slowly, with your mouth open wide, as you feel yourself relax.

Step Two Picture yourself in a safe, nurturing, comfortable place, and settle in. Breathe.

Step Three Think of a time when you have felt anxiety around eating—alone in a restaurant, in front of others, when you didn't like the food, when you felt full but continued eating, when someone made an unkind comment—and notice the physical and emotional feelings that arise in you. Breathe.

Step Four Follow the emotional thread of feelings from another time when those same feelings have surfaced in you, perhaps in a different circumstance and for different reasons. What was the occasion? Were you responding to someone else's behavior? Whose voice do you hear? What are they saying to you? Breathe.

Step Five What do you know about that other person, which may give you insight and perhaps even compassion into their circumstances? While it may not justify their behavior, does it explain it? Can you find a reason to forgive them for how they treated you? Can you find a way to forgive yourself for your own harsh self-judgment? Breathe.

Step Six When you feel ready, open your eyes. Take a moment to write in your journal what came up for you during this exercise. Include what you have realized and how you feel. Might you have a gentler sense of the other person and of yourself? What can you let go of? Breathe.

Macaroni and Cheese

MAC AND CHEESE INGREDIENTS

8 oz gluten-free elbow pasta
    (Tinkyada brown rice pasta)

2 tbsp butter

1 tbsp arrowroot

Salt to taste

Dash white pepper

1½ cups water

¾ cup full-fat coconut milk

10 oz sharp cheddar cheese

¾ cup more cheese for topping

COOKIE INGREDIENTS

3 cups almond flour

1 tsp baking powder

1 tsp cinnamon

½ cup coconut oil (melted)

¾ cup honey

3 tbsp maple syrup

2 tsp vanilla extract

3 eggs

2 cups peanut butter

A healthier twist on two classic comfort foods

DIRECTIONS

Preheat oven to 375 degrees.

Cook pasta as directed on package. While pasta is cooking, place cheese, water, coconut milk, arrowroot, butter, salt & pepper in the blender, and blend until smooth. Heat a medium saucepan. Add cheese mixture and cook for 7 minutes on medium heat, stirring constantly. Stir pasta into sauce and transfer to baking dish. Top with more cheese and bake until cheese is golden brown. Serve hot.

Peanut Butter Cookies

DIRECTIONS

Cream peanut butter, coconut oil, honey, maple syrup in medium bowl until smooth. Add eggs, one at a time, and beat for about 1 minute. Combine dry ingredients in small bowl, and then slowly add them to the wet ingredients until blended.

Drop spoonfuls of dough onto lightly greased cookie sheet, and press top gently with fork to add shape. Bake at 350° for 10 minutes, or until edges are browned.

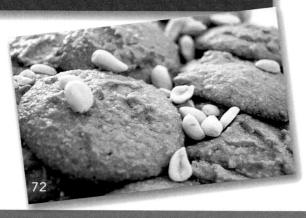

72

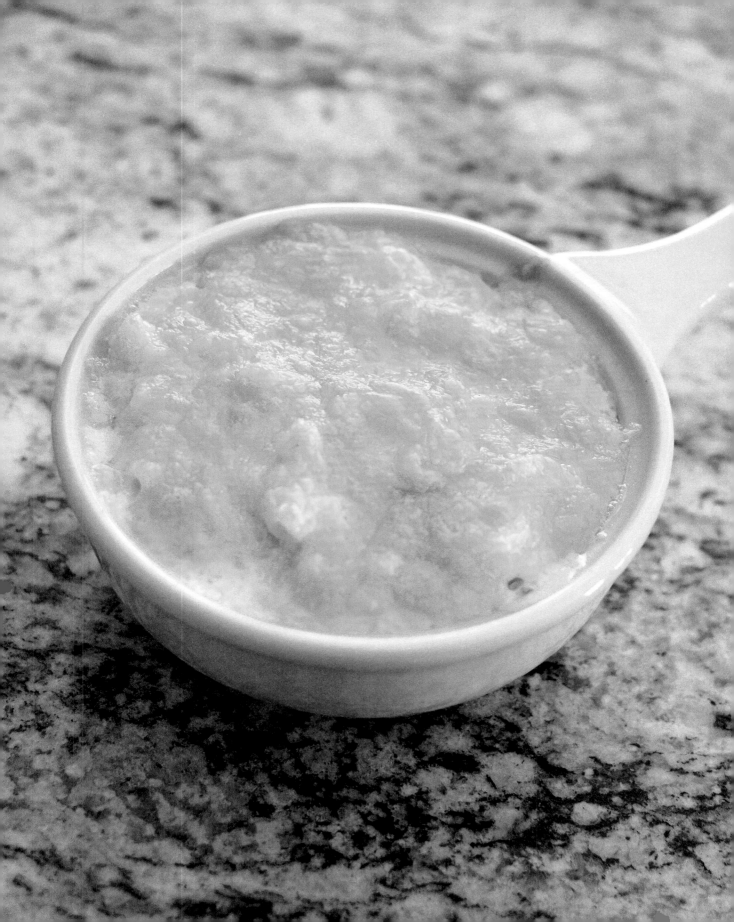

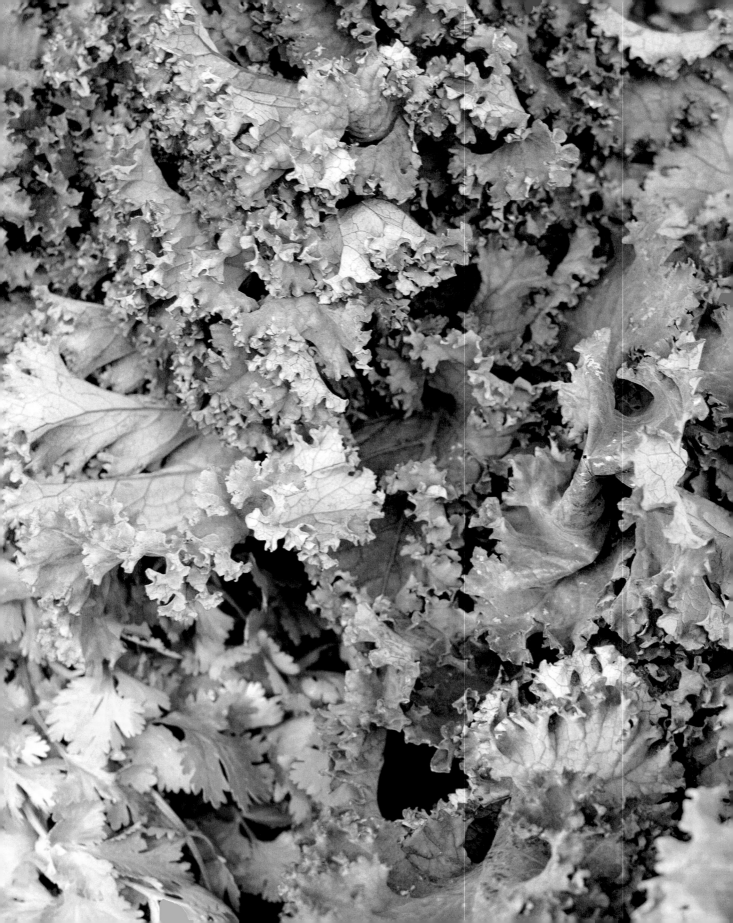

8

Conscious Choices

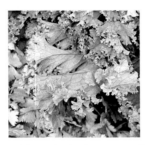

Just because we understand the importance of eating well doesn't mean it's easy. My neighbor decided, as part of her plan to eat healthier and lose weight, to stop buying double-dip chocolate ice cream bars and replace them with a fat-free version. Trouble is, while the fat content went down, as we now know, the sugar content went up to compensate for taste. Although the bars were low-fat, they actually carried more calories than the high-fat version. Contrary to her goals, she gained weight.

Upon the advice of her sister, another friend of mine replaced the banana in her morning protein shake with organic blueberries. Without making any other changes to her diet, she lost weight. Surprised, having assumed that bananas, as long as they were not cradling a hot fudge sundae, were good for her, she decided to investigate. Packed with potassium, bananas do have nutritional benefits. However, they also have a significantly higher-calorie density than other fruits, such as berries.

Calorie density, sometimes called energy density, measures the number of calories per pound in food. Understanding the difference can help us steer away from food choices that fill us up but don't nourish us and, instead, focus on foods that will provide the nutrients we need while helping us balance our blood-sugar levels, avoid cravings, and maintain a healthy weight. We see how relevant this is when we compare the different calorie densities (CD) in foods of the same category, such as fruit: bananas (CD 420), apples (CD 270) and berries (CD 140), or grains, as when considering oatmeal (CD 280) versus sourdough toast (CD 1,240) for breakfast.

High-energy foods, which have a low-calorie density, actually give us energy rather than robbing us of it. The more energy we have, the more efficiently we metabolize our food, the better we feel, and the more motivated we become to participate joyfully and productively in life. Think about how you feel after consuming a bran muffin or a stack of pancakes or a piece of layer cake. Now ponder the kind of get-up-and-go you would have after a fruit-and-vegetable smoothie, a garden salad or a piece of grilled salmon with a side of broccoli. Most likely, physically satisfied, comfortable and ready to move. Here are a few more foods and their CD values (more detailed information is available at www.cdc.gov/nccdphp/dnpa/nutrition/pdf/r2p_energy_density.pdf). These numbers are based on grams converted to pounds.

Cabbage 141	Brown Rice 504	Flour* 1653
Cantaloupe 154	Quinoa 545	*(white, wheat, unbleached)
Kale 222	Black Beans 599	Sugar 1757
Raspberries 236	Eggs 649	Walnuts 2969
Blueberries 259	Chickpea 745	Coconut Oil 3913
Sweet Potato 418	Steak 1017	Salmon 4095
Corn on the Cob 495	Buckwheat 1557	**Source:** www.cdc.gov

When we feel tired or we lack energy, we run the risk of making poor choices. Conversely, when we feel light, uplifted, energetic, we tend to make more conscious choices that benefit all areas of our lives. So, in terms of our nutrition, we want to get to the point where we are consciously, purposefully making positive choices instead of destructive decisions. When we choose foods that nourish us, that create the highest vibration and give us the most energy, we won't have room or even desire for the foods that don't.

Some people get up and go to the gym without question, or prepare a nutritious breakfast as part of a decision that's already been made. Others debate whether to get up and lace on those shoes or hit the snooze button; they put food in their mouths before considering its nutritional value or how it will support their morning activities. Both bear the consequences of their choices.

I have a friend who gets up early every morning without fail, and goes to the gym. She works out hard, in a variety of fitness modalities, and comes home two hours later, feeling invigorated, strong and appropriately hungry. Once she gets home, instead of making conscious choices about what to feed herself, instead of waiting to prepare a nutritious meal, she grabs a handful of chocolate-covered almonds, finishes the kids' toaster pastries, or sneaks a couple forkfuls of leftover chocolate cake. As she hops in the shower to get ready for work, she realizes she is now too full to eat something nutritious. Despite all her hard work at the gym, she is overweight.

Moreover, by 10 a.m., she starts feeling sluggish as she sinks into a sugar slump and becomes the colleague at the conference table who can't keep her eyes open.

Most conversations about eating for optimal weight focus on what not to eat. We call such food plans *diets*, which has become a dirty word, a depressing and usually temporary practice that devastates our social life as we can no longer attend a party without temptation or figure out what to order from the restaurant menu. Rather than focusing on deprivation, what if we turned our attention to what we can and should and want to eat? This is how we begin to nurture a healthy relationship between our body and food. As we train ourselves to be physically and emotionally attracted to supportive versus destructive eating habits, we will begin to crave the feeling of vibrating at a higher frequency, of operating at a higher metabolic rate, of feeling energetic and vital.

As Don Quixote said to Sancho Panza in "The Ingenious Gentleman Don Quixote of La Mancha," by Miguel de Cervantes Saavedra, "The health of the body is forged in the workshop of the stomach." It is in our core that we develop strength and generate our personal power, enabling us to focus, make clear decisions. We understand who we are as creative, loving, patient, purposeful individuals. In this state, we learn to identify and trust our own intuition.

This is the place where we feel aligned in every aspect of our lives, where we feed our bodies and nourish ourselves in all ways. Our health, our vitality, as a promise to ourselves, gives us an opportunity to live the highest experiences of life.

Goal

Develop a conscious awareness and accountability for what we're actually eating.

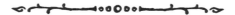

Step One   Select a notebook that will become your food journal. Make sure it appeals to you—the size is right, it has narrow lines, wide lines, no lines. Decorate the cover, make it yours.

Step Two   Using the Food Planning worksheet at right or a format of your own design, keep a daily log of what you eat, how much you eat, when you eat, why you eat and how you feel, physically and emotionally, afterward.

Step Three   Go to your neighborhood grocery store. Select any item from the shelves that you would normally buy. Read the label. Notice how many grams of fat, of sugar, of carbohydrates it lists. The American Heart Association says the maximum amount of added sugars we should eat in a day is:

- Men: 150 calories per day (37.5 grams or 9 teaspoons)
- Women: 100 calories per day (25 grams or 6 teaspoons)

How does your day add up? Reflect on your food choices in regards to both sugar consumption and calorie density.

Breakfast

Date	Breakfast	Breakfast	Breakfast	Breakfast	Breakfast	Breakfast	Breakfast
Protein							
Grain (optional)							
Fruit (1 serving)							
Fat (1 tsp)							
Other (optional)							

	Lunch	Lunch	Lunch	Lunch	Lunch	Lunch	Lunch
Protein							
Grain (if not eaten at breakfast)							
Vegetable (1 serving)							
Vegetable/Salad (1 serving)							
Fat (1 tsp)							
Other (optional)							

	Dinner	Dinner	Dinner	Dinner	Dinner	Dinner	Dinner
Protein							
Grain							
Vegetable (1 serving)							
Vegetable/Salad (1 serving)							
Dressing (2 Tbs)							
Fat (1 tsp)							
Other (optional)							

Artichoke and Asparagus Frittata

INGREDIENTS

1 tbsp extra virgin olive oil

6 large eggs

White cheddar cheese

Salt and pepper to taste

8 oz bag artichoke hearts

1 bunch fresh blanched asparagus
    (tender but still crunchy)

A tender egg frittata with fresh, nutritious vegetables

DIRECTIONS

Preheat oven to 350 degrees.

Whisk eggs in large bowl. Sprinkle with salt and pepper.

Mix 2 tbsp shredded cheese into eggs. Heat oil in medium-sized, nonstick, ovenproof skillet over medium-high heat. Add artichokes, asparagus, and red peppers to skillet, and stir for 2 minutes. Add eggs and stir to blend.

Reduce heat to medium. Cover and cook until eggs are almost set, about 5 minutes.

Sprinkle with more white cheddar. Transfer frittata to broiler. Broil just until set in center, about 1 minute. Using rubber spatula, loosen edges of frittata and slide out onto serving platter. Serve warm or at room temperature.

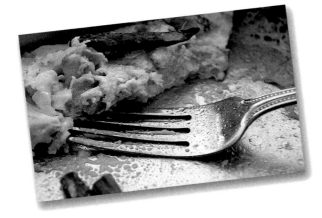

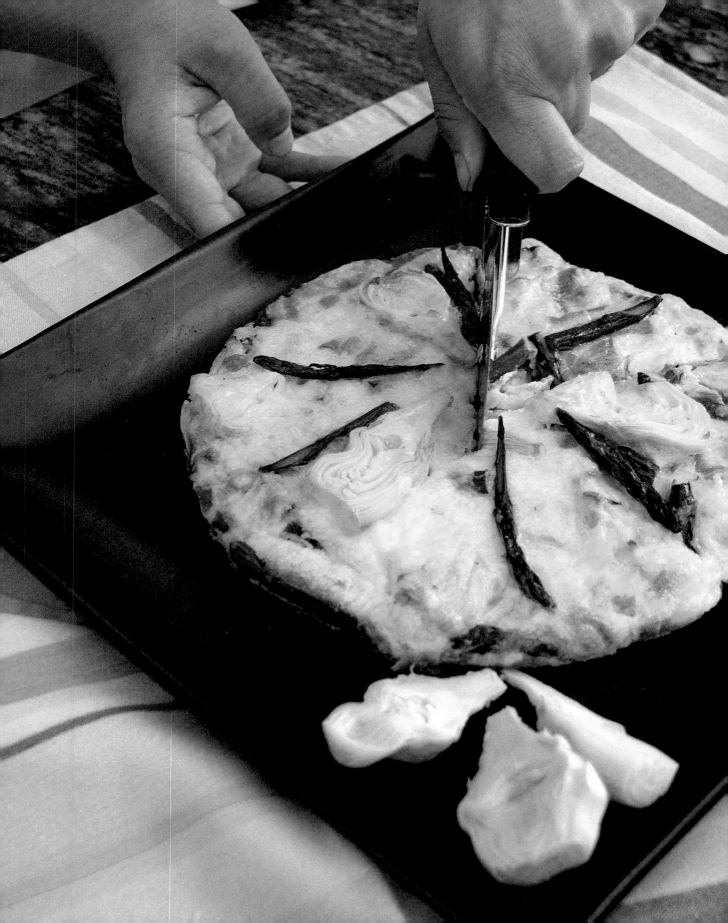

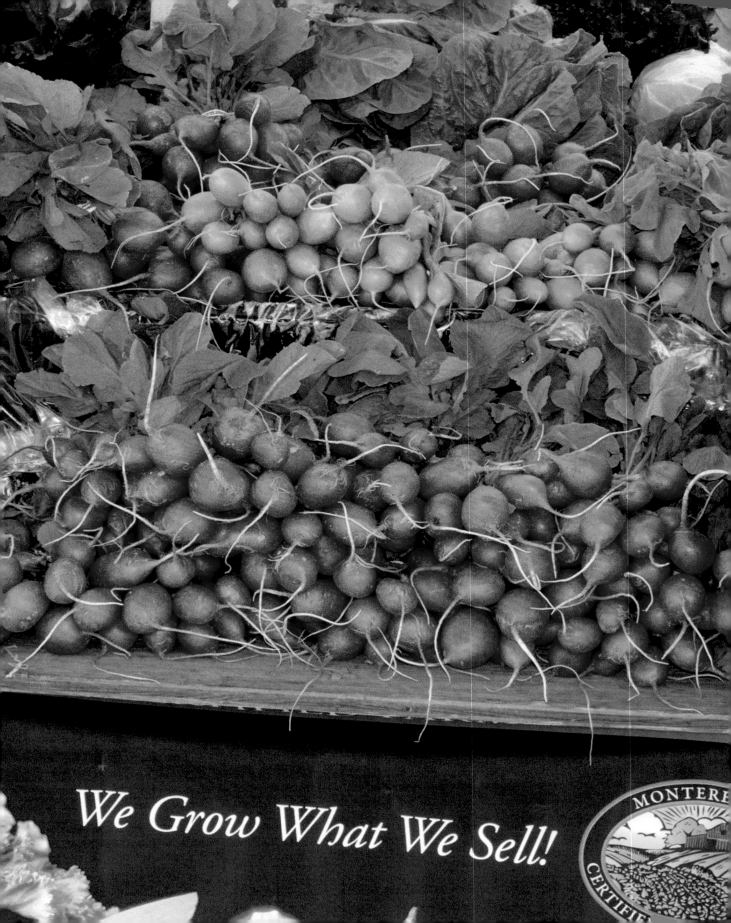

We Grow What We Sell!

It's Not Your Fault

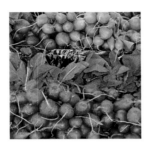 The most exciting part of my journey toward physical and emotional recovery from living with disordered eating habits and resulting weight issues came after I spent considerable time coming to understand the impact of my life experiences on me—and those of others on their lives—and I began to look forward.

Once I understood my present and my future did not have to depend on my past sense of self, that I could learn and apply important lessons to how I want to live and nourish myself now, I felt encouraged, excited, even.

Yet I've also learned that there is wisdom to be pulled from my past and, even further back, from preceding generations, which can be applied to what I'm learning now. Particularly when I look to a kinder, simpler lifestyle that came before the era of processed, packaged, preserved foods so many of us are serving ourselves today.

A couple of generations back, when my grandmother was in the kitchen, she made sure her family ate heartily and well. She'd pull a pot roast, meatloaf, or roast chicken from the oven, flanked by baked potatoes and carrots, or she'd add a serving of broccoli. She'd slice crusty, warmed bread she'd baked earlier in the afternoon, and nestle it within the folds of a cloth napkin tucked into a silver basket that had been her mother's. For dessert, she'd serve slices of dark chocolate cake she'd made from a family recipe, or maybe a dish of fruit cobbler with a scoop of vanilla bean ice cream churned over the weekend.

Everything was fresh and from scratch; nothing came in a box. There were no preservatives, no added hormones, no dyes, no additives of any kind. Grandma's only secret ingredients were a pinch of cinnamon in her stew, and a tablespoon of fresh-brewed coffee in her chocolate frosting.

Her husband came home from the office, and her children scurried in from school or sports or some game they were playing out on the sidewalk. They took their seats, held hands, said grace, and passed their plates.

No one complained, no one asked for something else, and no one had seconds. And no one was overweight. They appreciated and enjoyed what they ate and each other, as they took turns sharing the events of their day. I believe there was something special and meaningful about those ritualized meals. Here was a family coming together at the end of their day, to commune with one another, taking the opportunity to connect, and to nourish themselves and their most significant relationships.

The Institute for Integrative Nutrition® (IIN) teaches us this family was being nourished by more than their meal. They were enjoying a balance of what they call "primary foods™," which focuses on everything in our lives that "feeds" us besides food—relationships, spirituality, career, exercise, purpose. Maybe this is what people really mean when they talk about "soul food." And all this time I just thought it was mac 'n cheese.

Essentially, we are broadening the definition of nutrition as we look at all those things that give us the energy we need to thrive. Even in Abraham Maslow's introduction of his "hierarchy of needs," in his 1943 publication of "A Theory of Human Motivation" for *Psychological Review,* the psychologist placed food, water and air at the most basic level of need. Yet in ascending order from there, he acknowledged the importance of safety, love and belonging, esteem and self-actualization as essential life motivators.

All these years later, I still remember the exhilaration of marching in my white boots as a majorette in front of the band, twirling my baton in figure eights, tossing it into the air, and catching it in a continued spin. It was physical exertion and skill, pride and achievement, and just plain fun, all set to the invigorating rhythms of the likes of John Philip Sousa. That's a big helping of primary food™.

A client of mine told me how she found herself sinking into sadness at the loss of a friend, followed by the solace of a sedentary morning, supported by overeating. Until she decided to get up and out of her grief and go to her Zumba dance class. There, among friends, as she danced and breathed and got her "salsa on" to Latin rhythms, she felt joy and exuberance for the duration of the class and on into the afternoon.

These are examples of primary foods at work, nourishing our heart and soul, putting us in position to navigate the rest of our lives. This is about creating balance, so actual food doesn't have to assume complete responsibility. THIS IS BIG.

When all forms of nourishment; our relationships, spirituality, physical activity and careers or other purposeful pursuits are aligned, food loses focus. Think of all the times, particularly when you were a child, but even now, when you have gotten too absorbed in something to remember to take time to eat something. While this may or may not have been advisable, depending on your caloric needs, it does point out that we are nurtured and sustained by more than food.

According to IIN, we crave more than food, as we hunger, in varying degrees at various times, for play, touch, romance, intimacy, love, belonging, achievement, success, art, music, self-expression, leadership, excitement, adventure, spirituality and chocolate. When these primary needs are satisfied, chocolate tends to drop off the list. The extent to which we can incorporate these elements into our lives has a lot to do with how enjoyable and worthwhile, how gratifying our lives feel.

Chapter 9 Exercise for Positive Action

Goal

By better understanding the *Circle of Life, A Balancing of Primary Foods™*, we can discover which primary foods we are missing, and how to infuse joy and satisfaction into our lives. What does your life look like?

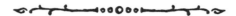

PART ONE

Step One   On the blank chart on page 89, place a dot on the line in each category to indicate your level of satisfaction within each area. Place a dot at the center of the circle to indicate dissatisfaction, or on the periphery to indicate satisfaction. Most people fall somewhere in between.

Step Two   Connect the dots to see your personal Circle of Life.

Step Three   Identify imbalances. Understanding that 100% personal satisfaction lies at the edge of the circle, determine where to spend more time and energy to create better balance in your life.

PART TWO

Step One   On a separate sheet of paper, list 3 to 5 life categories you listed closest to the edge of the circle; hence they reach almost 100% satisfaction.

Step Two   For each category you listed as closest to personal satisfaction, list the personal resources you used to get there. Perhaps it was the amount of time or attention invested, or perhaps focus, determination, passion, commitment, decisiveness or other skills. You will begin to notice you employed many of the same resources for each category.

Step Three List 3 to 5 life categories you plotted closest to the center of the circle, indicating you are least satisfied. To help usher these categories toward personal satisfaction, take those same resources you listed in Step Two, and consider how you might apply them here. This will ignite your plan to Balance Your Primary Foods™, moving you closer to a balanced, healthy life.

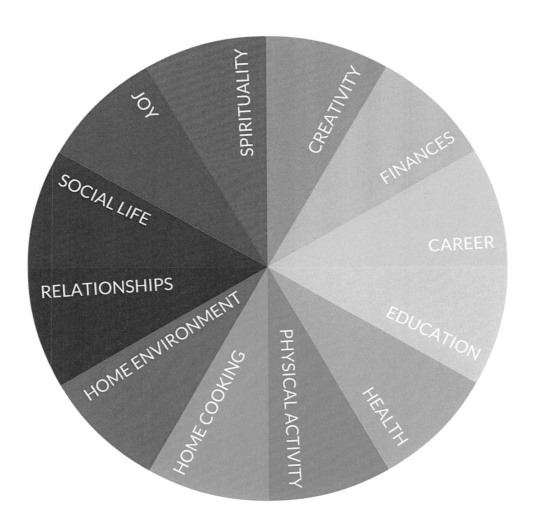

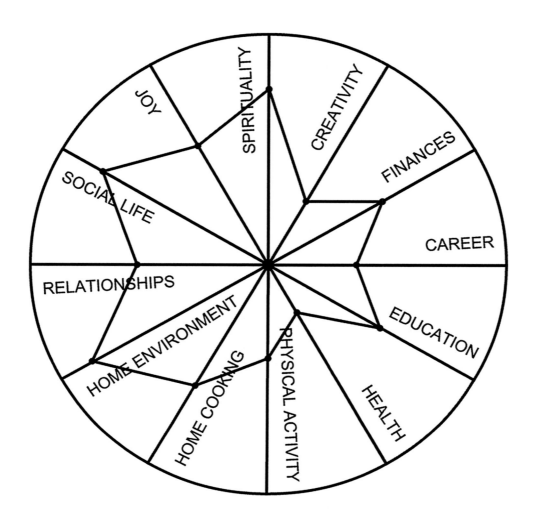

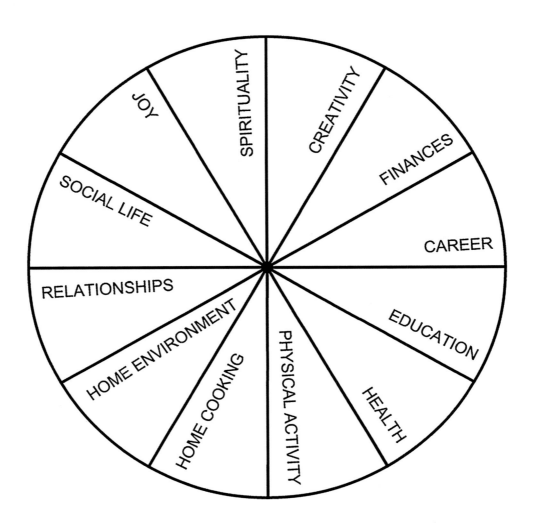

Two Smoothies and a Shake

GREEN SMOOTHIE INGREDIENTS

2 cups spinach

1 cup cucumber

1 cup frozen mango

1 cup frozen pineapple

3 mint leaves

2 cups water

MANGO VANILLA SMOOTHIE INGREDIENTS

2 cups frozen mango

½ tsp vanilla extract

1 ½ cups unsweetened coconut milk

1 tbsp chia seeds (optional)

HEMP PROTEIN SHAKE INGREDIENTS

3 tbsp hemp protein powder

1 tsp flax seeds

1 tsp chia seeds

1 tsp cinnamon

1 tbsp raw unsweetened cocoa
   powder

1 frozen or fresh banana

2 cups coconut milk or almond milk

All fresh-tasting and packed with powerful nutrition

DIRECTIONS

Place ingredients for each smoothie in a blender and blend until smooth.

(If using chia seeds for the Mango Vanilla Smoothie, mix them in quickly after blending. Enjoy smoothie right away, as chia seeds become gelatinous once they are wet.)

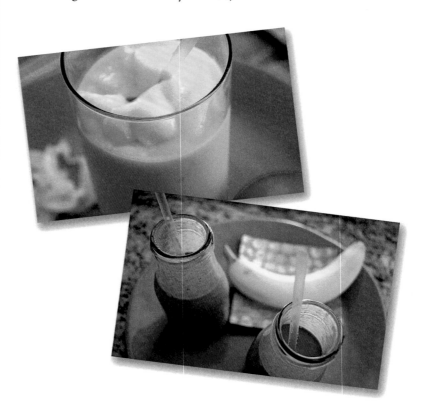

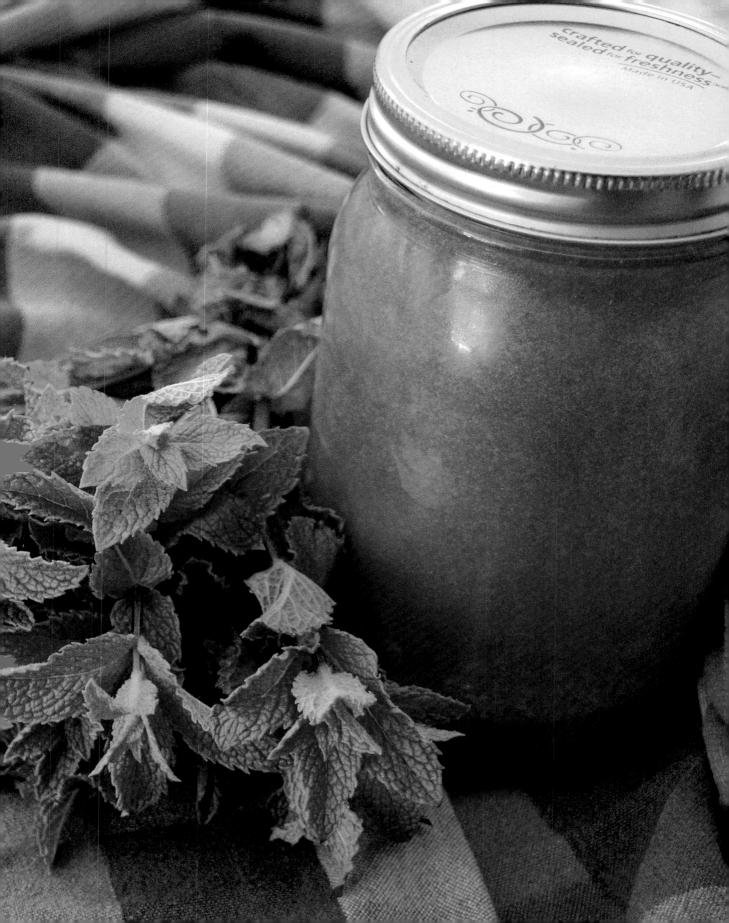

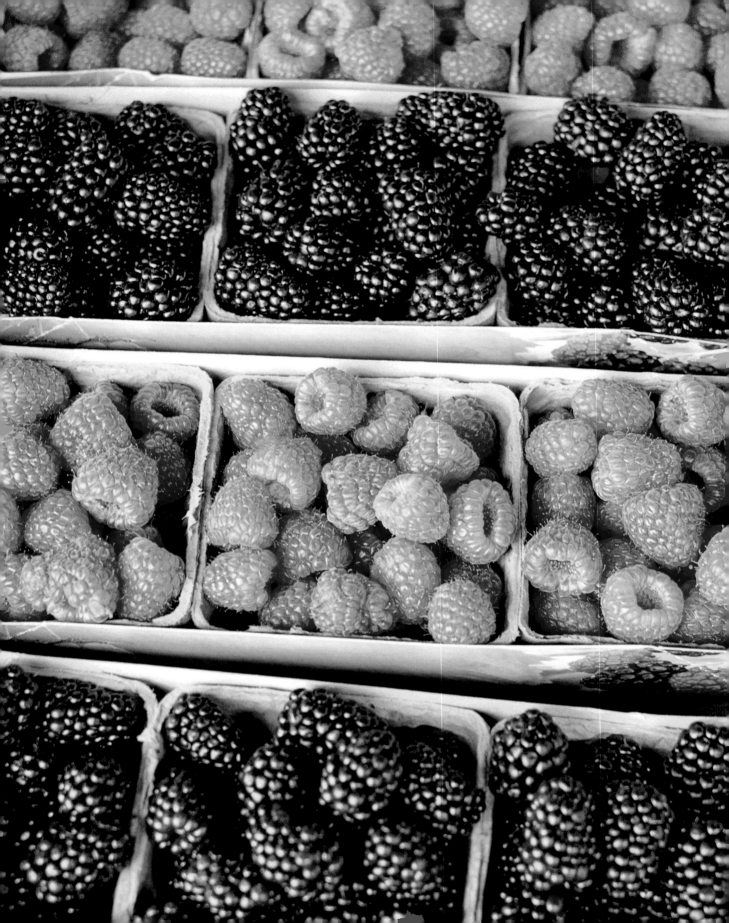

10

Feeding Frenzy

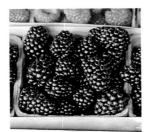 Much is made of the healing benefits of ice cream, especially when eaten right out of the carton. The go-to panacea for broken hearts, ice cream is cool and smooth and sweet, and goes down easy, filling the void left by unrequited love. Until it's gone. The carton is empty, and so are we, except for the icy inner chill and the nausea we mistook for heartache.

"Just a spoonful of sugar helps the medicine go down. . . in the most delightful way," sang Julie Andrews in Walt Disney's 1964 musical movie, "Mary Poppins." More than 50 years later, most of us still believe it.

The well-fed family has long been a symbol of abundance. Traditional postwar families, in particular, have been paragons of the "traditional family meal," complete with prayers, proper manners, polite conversation, and plenty to eat. The rituals, which in many families are now on the wane, were the glue that held the family together and gave us a sense of civility. But plenty, it turns out, was too much. And many American children have been fed a steady diet of myths for dinner. The starving children we heard about every time we dawdled at dinner would neither be fed nor honored because we finished everything on our plates. Dessert should never be a reward for eating vegetables. And the big news? The Clean Plate Club is no longer accepting new members.

Food can nourish—needs to nourish—our bodies. The right food, which contains the nutrients our bodies need, can help us feel better. But quick-fix food that feels good only when it's going down, can take us down further. With fake food, the kind that feeds our mind, our emotions, but not our bodies, we are fooling ourselves, believing it will help. With comfort food, that potatoes–pasta–cheesecake–chocolate-cream-pie kind of comfort, the soothing is only in the taste, texture and temporary satisfaction. After that, soothing slips into self-disgust for those who are overweight.

Just as my mother told me to go eat something, to make myself something sweet so I'd feel better, much of America has fallen prey to the sugar trap. Imagine an animal getting caught in a snare and finding it so seductive, he doesn't even try to get out. An animal will gnaw off its leg before letting itself die in a trap. We simply reach for another scoop of comfort. That's the power of addiction.

In the fall of 2014, filmmaker Stephanie Soechtig and journalist Katie Couric, following their investigation of the American Food Industry as it affects our weight and our disease states, released "Fed Up," a 90-minute documentary starring obese babies and chubby children and terribly overweight teens who are fat—and hungry. And the blame has been placed largely on the children as a lazy, sedentary, unmotivated, overfed generation that doesn't care. Look into the eyes of a child who can't see his shoes or bend down to tie them; into the expression of a child who eats alone at school, unchosen and unwilling to be seen eating; or into the anguish of a child who can't fit in his desk, participate in P.E., find someone to play with, or simply can't play. They care. I did.

Welcome to the new generation of overfed, undernourished youth.

In "Fed Up," we learn that, in two decades, 95% of all Americans will be overweight or obese if we don't do something about it, and that this is the first generation of children expected to have shorter life spans than their parents. We learn that by 2050, one in every three Americans will have diabetes. And we learn that it's all preventable. Once we know how. And if we do it. Knowledge is power only to those who possess it. And only to those who use it.

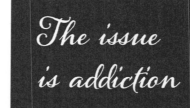
The issue is addiction

In the film, physician, scholar and author Dr. Mark Hyman, founder and medical director of the UltraWellness Center, says those who believe weight is an issue of personal willpower, of simply eating less and exercising more, are misguided. The issue is addiction. And, when 80% of the 600,000 food items in America are laced or loaded with sugar, he says, we don't stand a chance.

A 20-oz. coke requires a one-hour, 15-minute bike ride to burn off the sugar. And "sports drink" is a misnomer, particularly when a lot of the people guzzling 450 grams of sodium and upward of 25 grams of sugar in some of these beverages, aren't playing sports. We aren't going to simply exercise our way out of this. And plenty of people have learned they can out-eat even the most vigorous exercise routines. I'm one of them.

When I learned I'd been lied to, misguided by one of the most powerful, influential industries in the country—food—I began to realize, with a mixture of rage and relief, that many of my issues around eating and weight were not my fault. When I learned that research revealing that sugar is bad for our bodies went unpublished, I understood what it meant to fight a battle, uphill, in the dark, with the wrong weapons. I was angry. Unsure where to point it first, I decided to unload the gun, set it down and, armed with new information, wage a whole new kind of warfare by shedding light on hidden agendas dipped in sugar.

The food industry is filled with fallacies, baked into bite-sized pieces and stocked on grocery shelves in colorful boxes. Low fat doesn't mean low sugar; on the contrary, it usually means more sugar, added to enhance flavor in the absence of fat. The low-fat craze took America by storm.

In 2009, Dr. Robert Lustig, an American neuro-endocrinologist and professor at the University of California, presented a lecture called "Sugar: The Bitter Truth," about the deleterious effects of sugar on human health, which went viral when posted on YouTube. In his lecture, Lustig reminds us of Snackwells® low-calorie cookies, reportedly developed in 1992 by Nabisco's principal food scientist, Sam Porcello, which had 2 grams of fat less but 13 grams of carbohydrate more than traditional cookies, 4 of them, sugar. Such products gave rise to the social phenomenon known as the "Snackwell Effect," where dieters were motivated to eat more low-calorie cookies than they would have, traditional cookies.

Lustig refers to a book, published in 1972 by British physiologist and nutritionist John Yudkin, called, "Pure, White, and Deadly." It's not about cocaine, but some say it could have been since eating high-sugar foods, reportedly, lights up the pleasure centers in the brain the way cocaine does. The book was about sugar, and Lustig says he found it on-point. Although Yudkin's words were not popular upward of 40 years ago, "Everything this man said in 1972," says Lustig, "is the god's honest truth."

Lustig says we have neither admitted the mistake nor righted the ship. He says our food supply is adulterated, contaminated, poisoned, tainted on purpose by the introduction of fructose for palatability, as well as the removal of fiber. Some 50,000 years ago, he says, humans consumed 100-300 grams of fiber per day. Now, we consume around 12 grams. Why? Because fiber-filled food takes too long to cook and too long to eat, and has a short shelf life. Fast food, therefore, is fiber-averse. It can be frozen, shipped, cooked fast and consumed faster.

Some tell us it costs more to eat healthier. While I found it easier to eat poorly—there's not a lot involved in opening a package or microwaving a meal—I did not save money by eating fast food. Furthermore, I did not find that it costs more to purchase fresh produce; organic, grass-fed beef; and sustainable seafood. Yes, it does take a few more minutes to prepare, but I realized there is something inherently nurturing in the process of cooking quality food for my family. It looks better, smells better, tastes better, and it feels better going down.

Goal

Learn everything you can about the effects of sugar and
high-fructose corn syrup, and where they are lurking in your food.

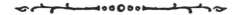

Step One   Watch any or all of the documentaries, "Fed Up," "Hungry for
Change," "Forks Over Knives" and "Food Matters."

Step Two   Take notes as you watch, paying attention to the information
that resonates with you, and the stories that inform and motivate you to make
changes in your own lifestyle and eating habits.

Information is power when you apply it. Take the steps to implement what you
have learned by reading labels, buying fresh, organic and sustainable, spending
more time at farmers markets than at big box stores, and making home-cooked
meals you can count on and enjoy.

Sprouted French Toast

TOAST INGREDIENTS

6 slices Sprouted Grain Ezekiel Bread

4 eggs

1 cup nondairy milk of choice
   (almond or coconut)

2 tbsp vanilla extract

1 tbsp cinnamon

1 tbsp maple syrup

coconut oil

BERRY SYRUP INGREDIENTS

2 cups berries

1 cup water

1 tsp vanilla

2 tbsp honey (or more if more
   sweetness desired)

1 tsp lemon juice

A Sunday favorite light enough to enjoy more often

DIRECTIONS

Whisk together eggs, vanilla, milk, maple syrup and cinnamon in a small mixing bowl. Soak bread well in the mix, coating both sides.

Heat nonstick skillet. Add a little coconut oil, and place bread onto hot skillet, turning occasionally to toast both sides. While bread cooks, heat berries and water in saucepan over low heat. Once they are halfway softened, add lemon juice, vanilla and honey, and cook until warm. Pour in blender and blend until smooth. Serve over French toast.

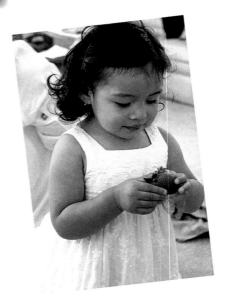

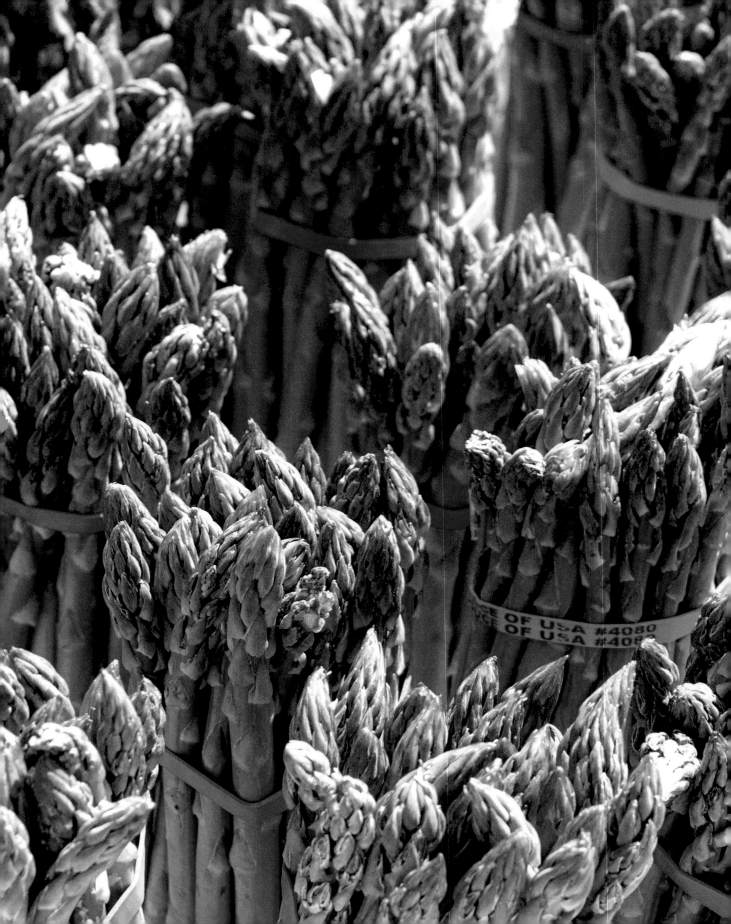

11

Good for the Gourmands

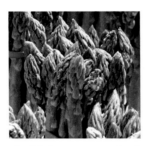

It blossoms across the plate like a flower, its petals soft, succulent, sticky. Slightly warmed before serving, it pulls apart easily, oozing caramel, icing, cinnamon and something secret. Paired with a sip of something steaming from a mug, it is as close to heaven as one can expect to get in this life. Sometimes she serves it with butter, but that might be considered "gilding the lily." Some people close their eyes.

A few of her friends try to use a knife or a fork, but then they don't get to lick their fingers. Which is part of the fun of my friend's signature cinnamon rolls.

Sometimes taste trumps, well, everything.

My friend will be the first to tell you, she has no problem with food. In fact, she loves it. *Loves* it. Not in an obsessive, has-to-have-it, all-consuming kind of love, but with the eye of an artist, the heart of a poet, and the passion of a chef. She appreciates food—the taste, texture, aroma, appearance—and she enjoys finding her ingredients at farmers markets, preparing meals for family and friends, experimenting with recipes, and watching it all come together as it cooks or bakes or grills or fries or freezes.

She's the kind of host whose large events and intimate gatherings appear beautifully catered, but they're not. She makes it all, herself. Monday-night dinner with the kids might be manicotti or mac n' cheese, chicken cordon bleu or chicken tenders, but no matter what, she's made it from scratch. And she savors every step of the experience, leaning in close to see the simmer, smell the sizzle. She licks her fingers, scrapes the bowl, and eats slowly, engaging all her senses to experience it fully and make it last.

Another friend would rather eat it fast and order seconds. She eats as much for recreation and entertainment as she does for the nutrients. Either way, she's nourishing something.

"I absolutely love to eat. I love food," she says, "I make my lunch as soon as I finish breakfast. By lunchtime, I'm already thinking about dinner. I plan parties around food, fully aware that celebrations often give me permission to indulge. My favorite way to travel is to eat my way through the city. My favorite way to spend an evening is cooking for friends, and the best part about Sunday is brunch."

Both of these friends are gormandizers, inclined to indulge in, or considered a connoisseur of good eating. And neither one has a problem with it. I read somewhere that binge eating is sometimes less about the amount consumed and more about how we feel about it. Those who are traumatized by what they eat or how much or under what circumstances. According to the Mayo Clinic, binge eaters consume unusually large amounts of food and, often, in secret. Just about everybody overeats on occasion, indulging in a second or third helping of a home-cooked or holiday meal. But those who eat copious amounts of food, with a compulsion to continue, and are consumed by embarrassment, shame or self-loathing, are binge eating. My friends are not. They are, quite simply, enjoying the indulgence of food.

And they are not alone.

Every spring, the Monterey Peninsula in California comes alive with thousands of gourmands, gussied up and eager to enjoy each other and the taste sensations prepared by some 75 celebrity chefs, paired with tastings from 250 acclaimed wineries. The Pebble Beach Food & Wine is known as the "premier epicurean lifestyle event on the West Coast." During this four-day indulgence, guests enjoy "intimate access to the pinnacle of culinary and wine talent" at wine tastings, cooking demonstrations and exquisite opportunities to taste.

This is but one of many culinary events around my area and across the country. And while guests are indulging, they are not overdoing it. They are sipping and savoring. They are tasting single bites of a carefully crafted appetizer, entrée or dessert, made with the finest, freshest ingredients by phenomenal culinary artists. They also are enjoying the music, the coastal view, the ambiance of the room, and fellow diners. This, my friends, is a pairing, not only of food and wine, but of primary and secondary foods. This is good food, good friends, good fun.

Think about when family and friends gather round the table to share a home-cooked meal. The sun, streaming through the window, or the candles lighting the night cast a glow on our faces as we take a moment to hold hands, to pass our plates, to feed our bodies with the fresh meal before us, and to nourish ourselves with communion and conversation. This is a perfect storm of primary and secondary foods.

Perhaps we can have it all, in good measure.

Chef Paola Mikes has a keen understanding of the importance of balance and the way to achieve it. She and her family enjoy good food, and one another, which is why she convenes them round the table for meals and why she began researching ways to rewrite the recipes of her family's favorite foods. She believed she could pair the primary nourishment of comfort foods with secondary nutrients inherent in quality ingredients to promote a happy, healthy family. And so, she has.

If you prepare your meals following Chef Mikes' recipes, will you lose weight? Perhaps, if you need to, but that really depends on how much you eat, how much you move, and how well you balance the other nourishing parts of your life.

Goal

This "Loving Behaviors" exercise is designed to open you up to the joys of primary foods™ in balance. This may be practiced by an individual or a couple. Either way, consider sharing your results with the people who love you.

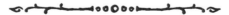

Step One   All you need is a piece of paper, a pen, and your present heart and mind.

Step Two   Make yourself comfortable in a place where you can write. Close your eyes, take in and release a slow, cleansing breath, and relax. Open your eyes and let yourself feel open to thinking and feeling.

Step Three   Consider an important loved one in your life. It may be your partner or spouse, your parent, your friend, your child. Fill in the sentence which is framed,

> When you _____, I feel loved.

Do this 5 to 10 times, each with a different answer. Examples:

- When you fold the laundry, I feel loved.
- When you take my hand in public, I feel loved.
- When you wink at me across the room, I feel loved.
- When you hug me, I feel loved.
- When you listen to me, I feel loved.

It is important that participants agree in advance to look one another in the eyes and receive the information without expressed emotion and without interruption. Know, as you share your responses with your partner, that what you report and what you hear are simply suggestions, an opportunity to learn about each other's needs and desires, without judgment, demands or expectations. This kind of genuine communication fosters an honest, openness in your relationship, developing a key primary source of nourishment. Complete your process by thanking one another for sharing.

It can feel soothing, satisfying, validating, even joyful to be heard, and often even more so to hear what your partner or parent or friend or child has to say to you. This is a wonderful way to develop empathy and compassion for yourself and others.

As psychotherapist Cristin DeVine says, "When you are not feeling enough love *from* someone, ratchet up your love *for* them."

Roasted Veggie Flatbread

GLUTEN-FREE CRUST INGREDIENTS

2 ½ cups almond flour

1 ½ cups arrowroot

2 tbsp olive oil

2 tsp baking powder

1 tsp garlic powder

1 tbsp Italian seasoning

2 tsp salt

½ tsp black pepper

⅔ cup coconut milk

4 large eggs

PIZZA INGREDIENTS

1 tbsp olive oil

4 cloves roasted garlic, finely
    chopped

1 ½ cups pizza or tomato sauce

10 oz Mozzarella cheese, sliced into
    ½-inch pieces (or shredded)

2 plum tomatoes, sliced

Roasted vegetables of choice

Handful of fresh basil

Pepper, to taste

*An artisan alternative to pizza with
a light, gluten-free crust*

DIRECTIONS

Preheat oven to 425 degrees.

Crust: Grease round pizza pan or rimmed cookie sheet with coconut oil. Mix all dry ingredients in medium bowl until well combined and set aside. In a separate small bowl, whip eggs with coconut milk and oil. Then add wet mixture to dry, and mix until well incorporated. The batter will be quite runny. Spread batter onto greased pizza pan and bake for 10 minutes. Remove from oven and set aside.

Pizza: Mix olive oil and chopped garlic in a small dish. Spread on top of crust. Top with pizza sauce, then Mozzarella cheese slices and roasted vegetables. Bake for 15 minutes or until crust is lightly browned, and cheese is melted. Remove from oven and top with fresh basil and pepper, to taste. Slice pizza and serve immediately.

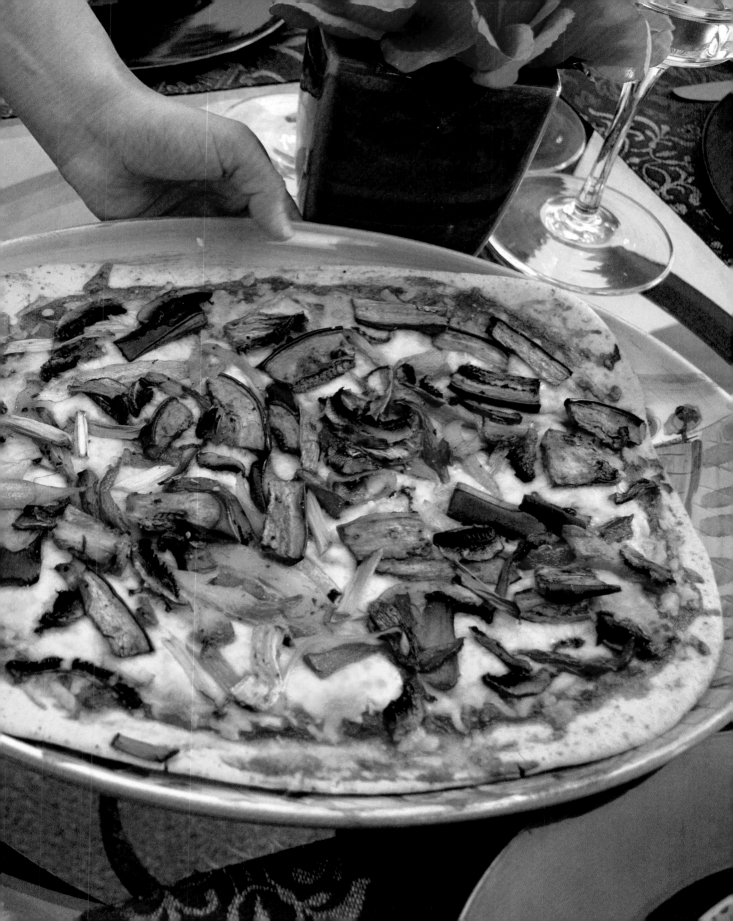

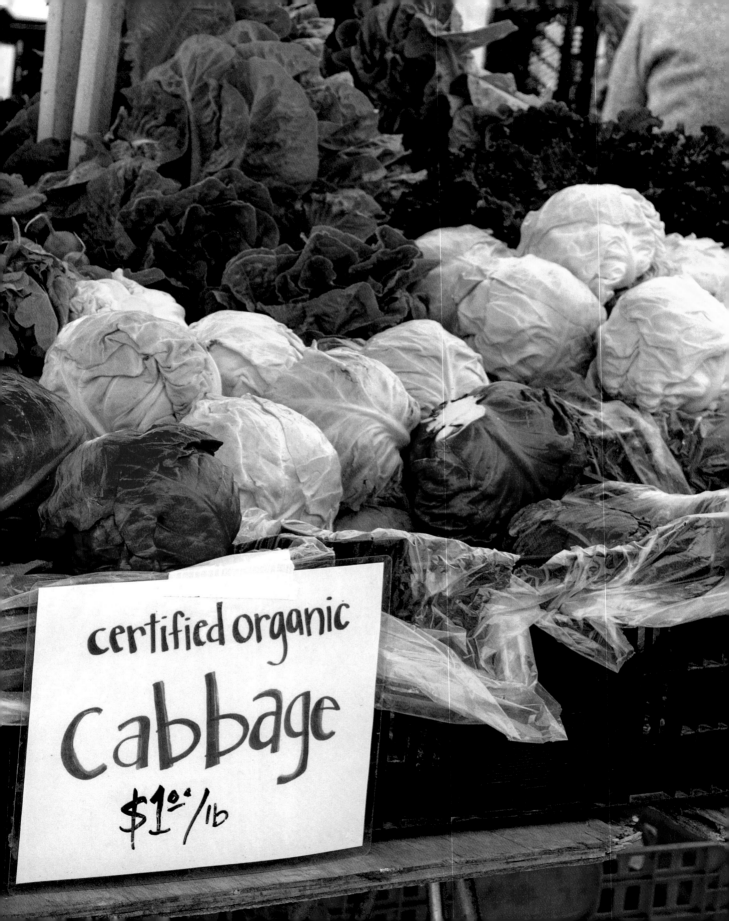

certified organic
Cabbage
$1⁰⁰/lb

12

Motivation and Resolve

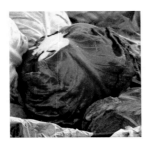

It was always hard to pore through the fashion magazines taunting me in waiting rooms, or leering at me among the other pieces of my mail, to study page after page of bare midriffs, toned arms, and cinched waists, just after I'd polished off another box of chocolates. Yet I continued to subscribe to the magazines and their impossible ideals because I love fashion and because it was like taking a walk on the wild side, venturing into a territory I had visited on occasion but had never taken up residence.

I was the kind of gal who hoped every morning, said a little prayer, even, that my clothes would fit; my pants would button, the patterns would match at the placket on my shirt or the wrap of my skirt. And I wondered what it must be like to wander through my closet, skimming along the hangers as I picked whatever I wanted to wear. In my fantasy, my questions were, "What's on trend or in season?" "How shall I accessorize it?" "What am I in the mood to wear?" Not, "Will anything fit me this morning?"

Even harder than studying fashion models in all their airbrushed beauty which, admittedly, gave me a bit of a pass, was reading article after article about women who had successfully shed 25 or 50 or 100 pounds, and had kept it off for five years. What was it about their character that had enabled them, not only to lose the weight but also keep it off? More importantly, what was the deficiency in mine that had allowed me to regain the weight every time? Why wasn't all the hard work, the sacrifice enough to keep me on the path once I'd reached my goal?

My friend Carolyn, who lost 120 pounds after that devastating trip to Disneyland, decided that, in making the life-altering decision to lose weight and get healthy, the individual has to identify in their own minds the reasons why they want to make changes. And they owe it to themselves to get clear about that.

"I think people know," says Carolyn, "when they get to that point, they need to do something. For me, it wasn't about getting into size-8 jeans; it was that I was a single mother, and I wanted to be there to raise my child. Then I realized that I, myself, wanted to have a more active, engaged life."

So don't approach your weight-stabilizing process thinking you have to diet or go without the things that previously gave you comfort. Look at it as seeking a different source of comfort, as a way to give yourself and your loved ones a true and lasting gift. You will find far greater comfort in something positive and real that will serve you well. The pint of ice cream, the chocolate, the cheese, the fries are temporary, fallacious, catastrophe-masked-as-comfort choices.

It's too hard to drop our source of comfort without replacing it. So we need to trade one form of comfort for another, healthier one.

For Carolyn, eating food in great quantities felt like a hug. But once she looked further into her life, she found more rewarding sources of comfort and inspiration in living a more active, engaged life with her friends and family. Once you realize that what you thought comforted you is not serving you well, and perhaps it never really did, it is time to make a change. Time to recognize that you want and deserve more out of life, and that it is within reach.

Information is vital to making a change. Yet we know we can arm ourselves with all the research and information in the world, understand it to the point where it becomes knowledge and still find that emotion, addiction, taste or habit can trump all of that. As a child, I would lick a lollipop until it made my tongue raw. And still, I would continue, until the candy was gone.

That's when we need a bigger, better, higher, source of motivation. Feeling better is a great motivator. And the anticipation of feeling better is a good place to start.

Only because we are creatures endowed with a temporal framework, with a sense of past, present and future, can we learn from our experiences, make changes in the moment, and anticipate—become motivated by—our future. It's the only reason we can farm the land, putting a seed in the ground, anticipating the sprout, and trusting it will grow, as it has, before. So we look forward.

Chef Paola Mikes found herself constantly looking back, aware that everything she had tried before to lose weight and maintain a healthy lifestyle for herself and her family, had either not worked or had not worked for long. As a chef, she knows a lot about food sources, food preparation, and healthy ways to feed herself. And, sometimes, she did it. So the idea of emotional, addictive, habitual or "it just tastes good" eating trumping knowledge of healthy eating resonated with her.

Until she saw the films "Hungry for Change," "Forks Over Knives," "Fed Up," and "Food Matters." These documentaries explore and expose the hidden villains, such as sugar, high-fructose corn syrup, and a slew of sugar substitutes that reportedly are contributing to food addictions, weight gain and the various disease states that can come from obesity; among them diabetes, heart disease, high blood pressure, hypertension, arthritis, cancer.

I will tell you; information that is startling enough can be a pretty powerful motivator. For Paola, the information changed her perspective on what she was doing, at the cellular level, to her body, and the impact it was having and would have on her health. Knowing she needed to do something to turn around her lifestyle and its deleterious effects, she joined IIN to learn how to nourish herself and those for whom she cooks, personally and professionally.

"And yet," she says, "I was still struggling. I knew what I needed to do every day in terms of eating and exercising, to be healthy. But I also knew I was surrounded by beloved people who didn't share my knowledge, my view, my efforts. And so, every time I was offered a sweet, every time my mom made a traditional Mexican dinner, I would cave. Every time.

"One can only be so strong in the face of temptation, day in and day out. I tried so hard, and yet I wasn't losing weight. If I did get on track and lose a little, my husband, who was not fully on board, would offer me a taste of something. One bite would lead to another and then another, until I wanted my own piece, and I gained back my own weight. I was so frustrated."

Paola wanted to be healthy and fit, and she actually knew what to do to get there. Because she couldn't bring herself to sustain her healthy eating habits, she felt horrible about herself, judging in herself a lack of self-discipline, conviction, self-control. On her more difficult days, she told herself perhaps she was not meant to be lean and healthy. Maybe she didn't deserve to feel good, to look good, to feel happy about herself.

"On better days," she says, "I put myself in a mind of acceptance, which was kinder to my feelings but not my body. Those stubborn 10 pounds tortured me as if they were 100 pounds. My clothes didn't fit, and those tight waistlines were a constant reminder of my failure. I was miserable. And I held myself responsible."

What Paola finally realized was that her knowledge of what to do to live a healthy, nourished life was not enough to help her sustain the practice. She also needed to create the right environment. She needed a support system to help her stay on track, to encourage her new eating habits. Particularly until she adopted her new lifestyle as her own, until it became second nature.

"Once I got my husband and daughter to buy into the idea of adopting healthier eating habits," says Paola, "it became easier for us to make it a lifestyle. My husband had gained 35 pounds eating traditional Mexican cooking, and he was unhappy with himself. Once he decided he wanted to do something about it, he lost the weight, fast. Now that I have made the changes I needed in my environment, I have come to a place where I feel good about myself. Even my parents and some of my friends have gotten on-board, which keeps me motivated to continue on this path. With time, it gets easier and easier for me."

For Paola, success came only after she made some decisions about her health and then followed up with the lifestyle and environment changes that would support her efforts.

"At the end of the day, armed with the knowledge I have," she says, "I know my well-being is up to me. I can't blame anybody else for my not eating well or not losing a desired amount of weight. No one can force me to eat but myself. But, I shouldn't torture myself, either. The better the choices I make, the better I feel, and so the easier it gets."

Through this process of self-discovery and lifestyle changes, Paola has been able to make peace with her body, her lifestyle and her health.

"It took me a long time to accept myself, to trust that I look the way I'm supposed to look," she says. "I am not choosing to eat a certain way just to look good; I want to feel good. This is the only body I have; I need to take care of it. Now, my husband constantly encourages me, and my daughter asks me to prepare healthy foods for her that make her feel so much better. I know we'll never go back to the traditional way we ate."

Learning what to eat is essential to nourish a healthy body. So is learning how. The time-honored tradition of gathering round the table for a hearty breakfast or a home-cooked dinner seems to have become the exception to a "grab-and-go" lifestyle. I understand and respect the dynamics of a busy day where we don't feel we have time to "slave over a stove" or linger over lasagna. Yet most of us are not aware of how much we suffer for it, sacrificing the benefits of our primary nourishment.

For breakfast, we sip Starbucks in the car, and throw down a donut or maybe a protein bar at our desk while paying attention to the road, the computer screen or the phone call. What we don't notice is what we are eating. The taste, the texture, how it feels going down or that it satisfies our hunger doesn't register. Our mind doesn't realize that we have eaten. So shortly, our brain, not our body, will ask us to eat again.

Moreover, we eat quickly, taking large bites or chewing like a squirrel to finish it fast and get back to business. It is over before we know it. Have you ever been piecing at something, a bowl of nuts, perhaps a package of M&Ms, and one time you reached for more, your eyes on whatever else you were doing, and you were surprised to find them all gone? This is called mindless consumption, a very unsatisfying way to eat.

When I was at The Meadows, they taught me to take time to eat, a daunting task for someone averse to making a ritual out of eating. I sat at a table, put a napkin in my lap, and used the table manners my mother taught me. Sometimes I lit a candle. I looked at my meal, breathed in the aromas. I filled my fork and slipped it into my mouth, savoring the food before I swallowed. I set down my fork between bites. And I breathed, taking in the experience. This ritual enabled me to consciously consume my meal at a pace that gave my body time to accept and acknowledge it. This time, when I felt full, I truly was.

Soon, I found myself eating less and enjoying it more.

This is aligned with a lesson Chef Paola shared with me. Whenever she ate while feeling stressed, no matter what she ate or how much or how little of it, she gained weight. Once she learned to slow down, to relax, and to manage her anxiety while eating, she lost a few pounds, without any other changes in her eating.

"If I felt overwhelmed and stressed," says Paola, "I took a couple of deep breaths before eating, to center my awareness and slow my cardiovascular system, so I could relax. Then I would chew longer and more slowly, finding myself at peace while I ate. Only by making these changes did I come to understand how stress was hindering my weight-loss goals."

I, too, have changed the way I eat; the choices I make, the reasons I feed myself, and the way I chew—more consciously, purposefully, slowly and for a longer period before swallowing. I have learned to set a lovely table, turn off the television, and pay attention to what I'm eating and those with whom I choose to dine.

I have shifted my focus from eating to feeding myself, finding nourishment in all aspects of the process, from choosing food at the farmers market, to preparing nutritious, delicious meals, to savoring it with someone I love and enjoy. This means there is no more shame associated with my eating habits and their effects.

This didn't happen overnight, nor did it happen all at once. Learning to nourish myself and teaching others to do the same is part of my life's journey. I now understand that the first part of my path is one many people take. As I have found and have chosen to take an alternate route along the way, it is my hope that I have helped you find your way, and that you are now headed in the right direction. I believe it is our God-given right to be healthy, to feel good about ourselves, and to know how to nourish ourselves in all ways. And to eat with grace.

Goal

Create an environment for yourself that stimulates and supports your efforts to comply with the healthy lifestyle you have chosen for yourself

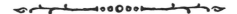

Step One   If you are seated at a dinner table, and the atmosphere is stressful, you feel tension at the table, or you feel uncomfortable—there is arguing, belittling, awkward topics of discussion, invasive questioning, pressure to eat something you don't want—honor your feelings and politely get up from the table.

Step Two   Leave the room, and find a quiet place where you can get grounded and re-center yourself.

Step Three   Close your eyes. Inhale, slowly spelling out the word R-E-L-A-X in your mind. Hold the air in for a few seconds and remain still. Exhale slowly, again, spelling out the word R-E-L-A-X in your mind. Do this until you have become physically and mentally calm.

Step Four   Return to the dinner table, relaxed, and with a clear mind, to resume your meal. Or, don't.

Chicken Tinga Tostadas

TOSTADA INGREDIENTS

2 boneless chicken breasts,
   cooked and shredded

5 Roma tomatoes diced

2 to 3 chipotle chilies in adobo sauce
   (add of all the adobo sauce)

1 medium onion, diced

2 garlic cloves minced

2 tbsp olive oil

MOUSSE INGREDIENTS

4 avocados

½ cup raw unsweetened cocoa
   powder

½ cup good quality honey

¼ tsp salt

4 cups mixed berries (thawed frozen
   mixed berries blend works best)

1 ½ tsp vanilla extract

⅓ cup coconut milk

Fresh, festive, tangy tostadas—with a special dessert

DIRECTIONS

In small saucepan, sauté onion and garlic in olive oil for about 4 minutes at medium heat. Add tomatoes.

In the blender, puree chipotle chilies and adobo, and add to tomato mixture. Stir in shredded chicken, and season taste. Cover skillet, reduce heat to low, and let simmer until most of the liquid has been absorbed. (About 15 to 20 minutes.)

EXTRAS

shredded lettuce   •   corn tostadas   •   guacamole   •   Mexican crema or sour cream   •   queso fresco (Mexican cheese)

Berry Avocado Mousse

DIRECTIONS

Place all ingredients in food processor or blender. Blend until smooth and creamy.

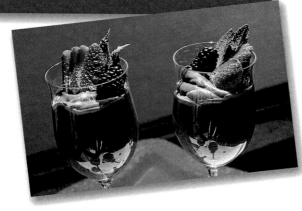

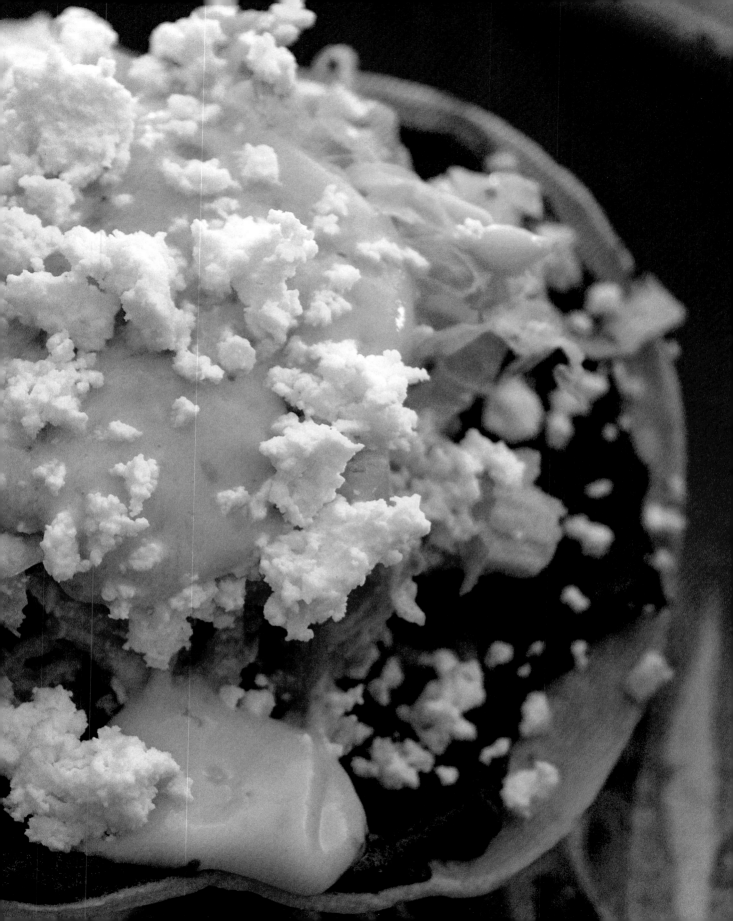

**You will know the truth,
and the truth will make you free.**
John 8:32

Epilogue

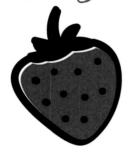

One of the most memorable messages I ever read in *The Daily Word,* so very many years after I had read that daily inspiration from Unity Church to my grandmother, regarded the freedom inherent in forgiveness.

In inviting readers to forgive ourselves and others, and embrace a new life, it said, "We are one with God, which means we are all good. Knowing this truth sets me free. In times when I am hurt or angry, I choose to see the good in others. This choice leads to forgiveness. As I release burden or blame, I am free to move forward in my life and embrace a new beginning."

I thought of various people in my life, from my earliest days to now, including myself, and the freedom I could feel to move ahead to my own health and well-being, if I could forgive. And so I have.

The message also said, "When I forgive, I wipe the slate clean. I replace feelings of anger, resentment, or fear with peace, love, and courage. These qualities reflect the truth of who I am and how I want to live. I am a free soul, unconditionally loved. As I forgive myself and others, I am at peace. I express love. I am courageous and strong. Through forgiveness, I am free of the past. I embrace a new life."

There is a reason they call it, "The Daily Word." These notions of cleaning the slate, of replacing dark emotions with light, of freeing myself by releasing blame, are challenges and opportunities I return to every day. It has become a practice, like any other skill whose mastery I endeavor. And the better I get, the better I become.

And so today, I am free and eager to look forward, leaning into my present and my future, with eyes open and curious, and ready.

And this newfound joy shows up in my life. The most exciting part about a recent Las Vegas conference I was planning to attend, besides what I hoped to learn during the seminars, was Las Vegas; the opulent environment of our hotel, the lights, the shows, the shopping. The most excruciating part about the conference was what to wear. More specifically, would anything fit?

A week before the conference, I pulled a selection of beautiful garments from the back of my closet, the tomb where clothes went either to die or await resurrection, depending on my weight. I hadn't worn these particular evening clothes in a few years, and I could feel, even as I fingered the fabrics and studied the styles, my emotions rise in a mixture of anxiety and hope.

I slid into the first piece, a long, shapely black dress I imagined perfect for evening events, and studied myself in the mirror. Once again, the dress did not fit. But this time, it was too big. This time, I was not.

Plenty of times I have thought I wasn't "there" yet in my efforts to live a healthy lifestyle and maintain the healthy weight that comes of that because I hadn't yet reached my destination (goal weight). Yet what I've come to understand is that I am there; I am on the right path, which is where I want to be.

If life really is a journey, then my goal should be to carry on along the highest and best possible route. And now that I have the knowledge I need to proceed, I can find my way.

I often think of the passage in Richard Bach's beloved book, "Jonathan Livingston Seagull—a story."

"Jonathan is met by two gulls who take him to a 'higher plane of existence' in which there is no heaven but a better world found through perfection of knowledge. . . In this new place, Jonathan befriends the wisest gull, Chiang, who takes him beyond his previous learning. . . The secret, Chiang says, is to begin by knowing that you have already arrived."

I am committed to making good, healthy choices for myself. Will I make less-healthy choices now and then? Will I, on occasion, cater to my cravings or indulge an emotion? Absolutely. But this time, I won't beat myself up for it. I may even allow myself to enjoy the moment. Then, as if merely having hit a speed bump in my path, I will get back on track and continue on my way.

So often, we learn about an idea, a concept, a suggestion, and feel encouraged, even hopeful. Yet we tend to take it in as something to contemplate instead of something to actually try out. I invite you to do both, to consider and practice the ideas and exercises I have shared with you, and then you can contemplate their value for your life.

Now that you have wandered alongside my journey, hopefully exploring your own along the way, I encourage you to share your own experiences, seek support or guidance through health coaching or perhaps a more expanded explanation of exercises and practices introduced within this book.

You are welcomed and encouraged to contact me through Advanced Health Coaching at **www.advancedhealthcoaching.com,** or **revgrace@icloud.com,** or by calling **831.644.9614**.

~ Rev. W. Grace Nicodemus

Chocolate Coconut Tart

SHELL INGREDIENTS

½ cup unsweetened shredded
    coconut

1 ½ cups almond flour

¼ cup macadamia nuts,
    finely chopped

2 tbsp coconut oil

¼ tsp salt

2 tbsp maple syrup
    or coconut nectar

GANACHE INGREDIENTS

1 ¼ cup full-fat coconut milk

12 oz chocolate, finely chopped
    (65% cocoa)

1 tsp vanilla extract

⅛ tsp coarse sea salt

TOPPING

½ cup unsweetened coconut flakes

Healthy eating has never tasted so indulgent

DIRECTIONS

Preheat oven to 350 degrees.

Tart shell: In food processor, pulse together almond flour, salt, shredded coconut and macadamia nuts until finely ground. In a saucepan, melt together coconut oil and maple syrup. Add to almond flour and coconut mixture. Pulse until coarse crumbs form (dough should clump together when squeezed with fingers).

Transfer dough to greased 9-inch tart pan with a removable bottom. Using your fingers, evenly press dough in bottom and up sides of pan. Bake in center of oven until golden and firm, about 15 to 20 minutes. Transfer to a wire rack to cool completely, at least 1 hour.

Spread shredded coconut evenly over sheet pan, and bake until lightly golden, about 3 to 5 minutes. Set aside.

Ganache: Place chopped chocolate in large mixing bowl. In small saucepan, bring coconut milk to a boil. Pour hot coconut milk over chocolate and let stand 1 minute. Stir until smooth and creamy. Mix in vanilla extract.

Tart Assembly: Pour chocolate into cooled tart shell. Lightly sprinkle with toasted coconut. Chill for at least one hour or until set.

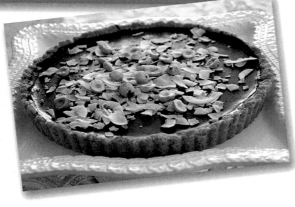

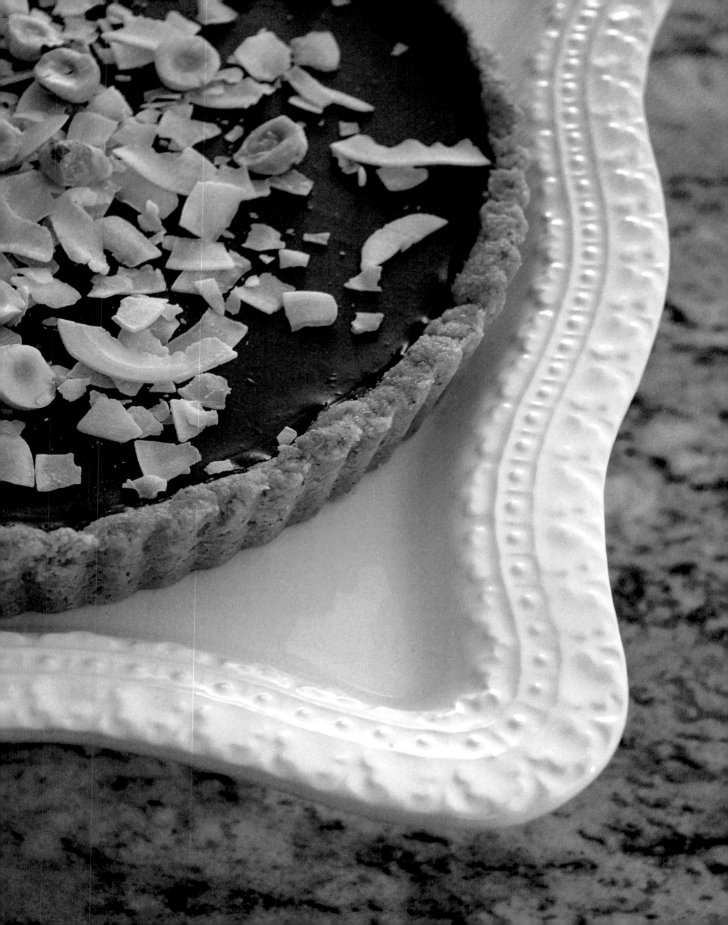

ABOUT THE

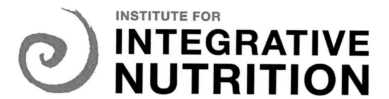

INSTITUTE FOR
INTEGRATIVE NUTRITION

IIN was established in 1992 by Joshua Rosenthal, whose mission is to play a crucial role in improving health and happiness and, through that process, create a ripple effect that transforms the world. What began as a small gathering of students in a rented kitchen, determined to learn about health and wellness through better nutrition, IIN is now reportedly the largest nutrition school in the world.

"This is an extraordinary time in medicine," says Mark Hyman, MD, founder of The UltraWellness Center, "because those people who have provided healthcare in the past, namely doctors, are not going to be the people who create health in the future. Those are going to be health coaches."

Through an innovative online "learning platform" that goes beyond philosophy to teach practical application of nutrition principles, IIN reports having provided training to more than 50,000 students in 122 countries.

"I think the success of programs like IIN," says Deepak Chopra, MD, "resides in the fact that they introduce very diverse points of view and are not rigidly attached to any one philosophy."

Yet the core philosophy presented by the school is that IIN was founded on two major principles: primary food and bioindividuality. Primary food™, by its definition, includes everything that fuels us beyond the food on our plate—relationships, physical activity, career and spirituality. When these are in balance, our life nourishes us, making what we eat complementary to our wellbeing. Bioindividuality™, according to IIN, is the principle that every person has unique dietary and lifestyle needs.

"One of the things that was important to me," said Rosenthal, "was to establish a school where people could develop a career within a year. Go out, earn money, see clients, and make a difference in the world. So many schools teach "ivory tower" theory. They understand how the body works but don't get training on how to talk to an individual to help them make a difference for themselves and their family. That's a crucial difference that happens in our school."

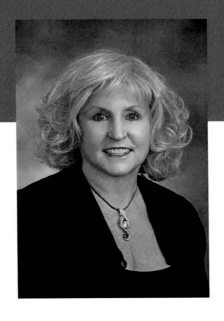

Rev. W. Grace Nicodemus

Trauma, followed by healing, creates a portal to the compassionate heart. Coupled with years of specialized training and reflection, The Rev. W. Grace Nicodemus comes from a place of knowing and understanding as she escorts her clients along their journey to recovery. A seasoned businesswoman in finance, securities and real estate, Rev. Grace shifted her career to client coaching and patient recovery as she effected her own process of healing.

With her bachelor's degree in Business Relationships and Psychology, along with her ordination as a Unity minister, and certification in Medical Hypnosis, Rev. Grace provides preventive medicine and health coaching to help patients and clients experience healthy, sustainable behavior changes. Working from a supportive, non-judgmental and empathic approach, she focuses on the mind, body and spirit, encouraging patients to listen to their inner wisdom to transform their goals and desires into action.

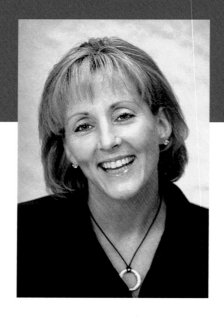

Lisa Crawford Watson

A fifth-generation Northern Californian, Lisa Crawford Watson belongs to one of three sets of twins in a large and dynamic family—at times, the source of her writing. With an undergraduate degree in Sociolinguistics from the University of California at Davis, a Master's degree in Education Administration from California State University, Sacramento, an postsecondary teaching credential and her Real Estate license, she has enjoyed a diverse career in business, education and writing.

A scion of storytellers, Lisa lives with her family on the legendary Monterey Peninsula, where her grandmother once lived and wrote. An adjunct instructor of writing and journalism for California State University Monterey Bay and Monterey Peninsula College, Lisa is a writer who specializes in narrative as she covers the genres of art & architecture, health & lifestyle, food & wine. She has published various books and thousands of feature articles and columns in local and national newspapers and magazines. In addition to fitness, fun and family, writing defines both who she is and what she does.

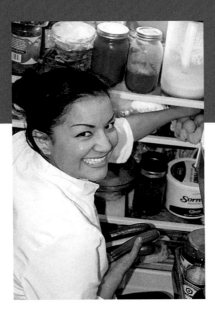

Chef Paola Mikes

Born in Oaxaca, Mexico yet raised in Northern California, Chef Paola Mikes grew up in a culture of food. She trained in her mother's kitchen, learning to cook traditional foods that were rich and tasty, to feed a large and hungry family. And everyone grew big on such compassionate cooking. She cooks differently now.

At the Monterey Culinary Institute, Chef Mikes learned to pair traditional cooking with a more sustainable style of food preparation. Upon graduation, she honed her skills as a chef on the legendary Cannery Row in Monterey and in several Carmel restaurants.

Soon she began to experiment, replacing corn oil, canola oil or lard with olive or coconut oil. Eliminating refined sugars, she shifted to honey or agave, and replaced white flour with almond or brown-rice flour. Spending more time at local farmers markets than at supermarkets, and choosing fresh, organic food over packaged, processed foods, Chef Mikes proved that healthy eating costs less, particularly in terms of the toll her traditional cooking took on the body.

List of Recipes

Resources

- American Heart Association. www.heart.org

- DeVine, Cristin, MFT, *Pathways to Wholeness Psychotherapy*. www.counselingcarmel.com.

- Macmillan. (1970). *Jonathan Livingston Seagull—a story,* Bach, Richard

- Disneyland, *Mickey's Toontown.* Anaheim, Calif.

- Fed Up. (2014). Katie Couric, Laurie David, fedupmovie.com

- *Sugar, the Bitter Truth,* (2009) Dr. Robert Lustig, president of the Institute For Responsible Nutrition. http://www.uctv.tv/shows/Sugar-The-Bitter-Truth-16717.

- *Food Matters.* (2008) Colquhoun, James and ten Busch, Laurentine, http://www.foodmatters.tv.

- *Hungry for Change.* (2012) Colquhoun, James and ten Busch, Laurentine. http://www.foodmatters.tv.

- *Forks Over Knives.* (2011) Virgil Films and Entertainment. www.forksoverknives.com

- Walt Disney. (1964). *Mary Poppins,* an American musical fantasy film adapted from the book of the same name by Travers, P.L.

• www.mayoclinic.org, *Binge Eating*

• Psychological Review. (1943). *A Theory of Human Motivation*. Maslow, Abraham.

• Rader Programs, Occupational Therapy, Rehabilitation Center, Counseling & Mental Health (Closed)

• *Institute for Integrative Nutrition*. (2015). Rosenthal, Joshua. www.integrativenutrition.com

• Francisco de Robles, publisher. (1605). *Don Quixote*. Saaveda, Miguel de Cervantes.

• Scottsdale, Arizona. (2015). *The Meadows Trauma & Addiction Treatment Program*. www.themeadows.com

• Unity Worldwide Ministries. www.unityworldwideministries.org

• Davis-Poynter, London. (1972). *Pure, White and Deadly*. Yudkin, John.

• *Shrinking Violet,* (1963). The Funny Company.